THE ANTI-INFLAMMATORY ACTION PLAN

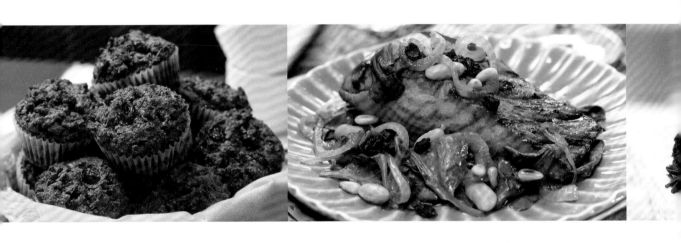

THE ANTI-INFLAMMATORY ACTION PLAN

Incorporate Omega-3 Rich Foods into Your Diet to Fight Arthritis, Cancer, Heart Disease, and More

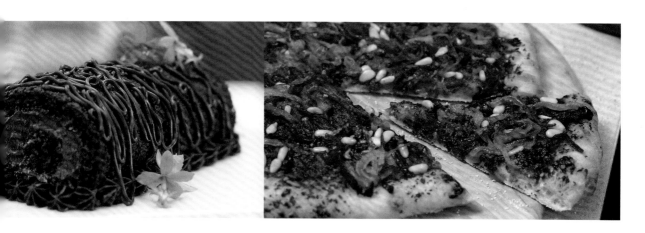

BARBARA ROWE
M.P.H., R.D., L.D., C.N.S.A.

&

LISA DAVIS
Ph.D., P.A.-C., C.N.S., L.D.N.

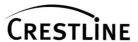

CRESTLINE

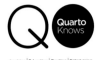

Brimming with creative inspiration, how-to projects, and useful information to enrich your everyday life, Quarto Knows is a favorite destination for those pursuing their interests and passions. Visit our site and dig deeper with our books into your area of interest: Quarto Creates, Quarto Cooks, Quarto Homes, Quarto Lives, Quarto Drives, Quarto Explores, Quarto Gifts, or Quarto Kids.

Text © 2008 Fair Winds Press

This edition published in 2019 by Crestline,
an imprint of The Quarto Group
142 West 36th Street, 4th Floor
New York, NY 10018 USA
T (212) 779-4972 F (212) 779-6058
www.QuartoKnows.com

First published in 2008 by Fair Winds Press, an imprint of The Quarto Group,
100 Cummings Center, Suite 265-D, Beverly, MA 01915, USA.

Crestline titles are also available at discount for retail, wholesale, promotional and bulk purchase. For details, contact the Special Sales Manager by email at specialsales@quarto.com or by mail at The Quarto Group, Attn: Special Sales Manager, 100 Cummings Center Suite 265D, Beverly, MA 01915 USA.

10 9 8 7 6 5 4 3 2 1

ISBN: 978-0-7858-3802-9

Book design: Emily Brackett/Visible Logic
Photography: Madeline Polss
Food Stylist: Dwayne Ridgaway

Printed in China

Previously published as *Anti-Inflammatory Foods for Health*.

The information in this book is for educational purposes only. It is not intended to replace the advice of a physician or medical practitioner. Please see your health care provider before beginning any new health program.

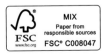

Contents

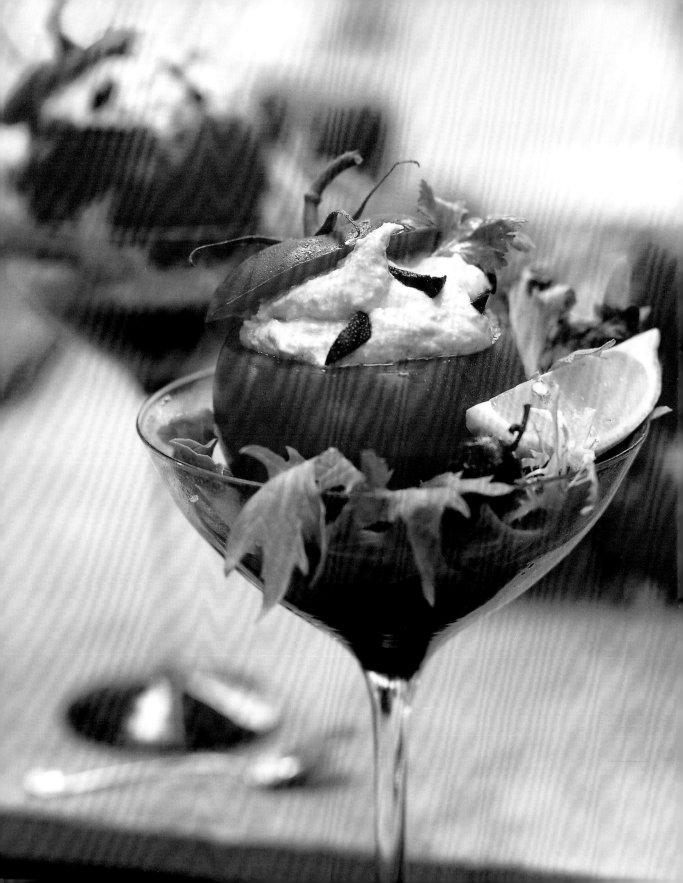

Introduction

Inflammation and Disease

Increasingly, we are becoming aware that inflammation underlies many of the world's most common diseases, even the process of aging. Clearly, inflammation is associated with such obvious inflammatory conditions as rheumatoid arthritis, but did you know that inflammation is a risk factor for developing heart disease and cancer, our most common killers?

Given this, shouldn't we all be trying to do something to reduce inflammation? One thing we all can do is to eat healthier foods—foods that help combat inflammation.

Let this recipe book serve as your guide to preventing or combating inflammation and improving your health through diet. The calorie-controlled recipes you will find in each chapter will not only help fight inflammation, but they will also help you control excess body weight—a major risk factor for inflammation.

OBESITY AND INFLAMMATION

Too much body weight is one of the clearest links between inflammation and disease. Carrying extra pounds, particularly around the middle of your body (abdominal obesity), is a risk factor for inflammation. The reason is that fat (especially abdominal fat) is metabolically-

Table 1: Health Conditions Associated with Inflammation

System	Health Conditions
Cardiovascular	High cholesterol or triglycerides, high blood pressure, stroke, sudden death
Endocrine	Type-2 diabetes, metabolic syndrome, nonalcoholic fatty liver disease
Pulmonary	Asthma
Gastrointestinal	Inflammatory bowel disease (e.g., ulcerative colitis, Crohn's disease)
Immune	Rheumatoid arthritis, multiple sclerosis, allergies, psoriasis, atopic dermatitis
Cellular	Cancer (especially breast, colon, and prostate)
Psychological	Schizophrenia, mood disorders (e.g., major depression)

active tissue. Metabolically-active fat tissue releases all kinds of inflammatory molecules into our bloodstreams, which travel to target organs, such as the heart.

Inflammatory molecules released by fat tissue don't affect just the heart, though. They affect the cells of all body organ systems, from the lungs, to the joints, to the central nervous system. They present as a number of different diseases, including cardiovascular disease (high cholesterol), asthma, diabetes or metabolic syndrome, rheumatoid arthritis, multiple sclerosis, and cancer, and they can even affect our moods. If you are suffering from any of the diseases listed in **Table 1** (see page 7), this nutrition and recipe guide may be of special benefit to you.

Often, these disease states arise from too much oxidative stress in the body as a result of all of this inflammation. All too often, a vicious cycle forms because too much oxidative stress also worsens inflammation. Oxidative stress also is a serious concern because it triggers the formation of free radicals. Free radicals change your body's cells in negative ways and make you susceptible to such illnesses as cancer and heart disease. If you consume too much fat (especially in the form of saturated fat, trans fat, and omega-6 fat), too much sugar, too many calories, and

are carrying too much extra body weight, you are likely to have too much inflammation and oxidative stress in your body **(Figure 1).**

Figure 1: The Formation of Inflammation and Oxidative Stress

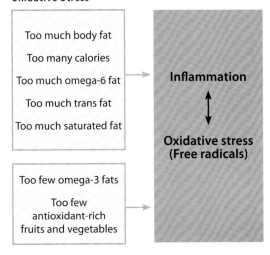

If you think you might be at risk for having too much inflammation, either because you have diabetes and high cholesterol or have a strong family history of heart disease, you can ask your doctor to order a special test called C-reactive protein. This is one of a number of chemical markers in your body that increase in response to inflammation. C-reactive protein levels are normally elevated acutely in response to injury. However, when levels of C-reactive protein are mildly to moderately elevated on a long-term basis, they set the stage for such chronic diseases such as cardiovascular disease and diabetes and tend to indicate that ill health effects are brewing.

The Role of Diet in Inflammation

There is a strong relationship between our Western diet and inflammation. Over the last century, food industry practices have changed such that we are increasingly exposed to inflammatory foods without our knowledge or understanding. Two of the main nutritional influences in the body that are inflammatory include the types of dietary fat we eat and the amount of highly sugared carbohydrates we consume.

Clear relationships exist between dietary patterns and inflammation. Some of the main staples in our diets are quite inflammatory: Sugar-sweetened soft drinks, refined grains, processed meats, and a low ratio of omega-3 to omega-6 fats are all associated with inflammation. Things we know that help to reduce inflammation include fish, vegetables, fruits, walnuts, olive oil, and even red wine. Let's take a closer look.

FATS IN OUR DIETS

The concept of "good" fats and "bad" fats is not new. But, as we continue to conduct research, more and more is learned about the role different types of fat play in our diets and health. **Table 2** provides an overview of the types of dietary fat.

Table 2: "Good" Fats and "Bad" Fats

Good Fats	Main Dietary Source
Monounsaturated	Olive oil, canola oil, peanut oil, almonds, avocados
Polyunsaturated	Vegetable oils (corn, soybean, safflower, cottonseed), fish
Bad Fats	
Saturated	Whole milk, red meat, butter, cheese, coconut oil
Trans	Partially hydrogenated vegetable oils, most margarines, vegetable shortenings, baked goods, commercially prepared french fries and onion rings

THE GOOD FATS
Polyunsaturated Fats (PUFAs)

There are two main types of PUFAs: omega-3 fats (linolenic acid) and omega-6 fats (linoleic acid). Both omega-3 fats and omega-6 fats are essential fatty acids (EFAs), meaning that while they are important and necessary, the body doesn't manufacture them so they must be obtained through our diets. That gives us an opportunity to choose our PUFA fats wisely and have some control over how much inflammation we introduce into our bodies through this dietary source. What we have learned through research is that fatty acids of the omega-6 variety have more inflammatory properties than the omega-3 type. Omega-3 fatty acids are therefore considered less inflammatory (or anti-inflammatory).

There has been a shift in the types of PUFAs in our diets over the last century—a shift toward more inflammatory fats. Before modern processing methods modified our diets to contain more processed foods, the ratio of omega-6 to omega-3 fatty acids was approximately 4:1. Today, the ratio of omega-6 to omega-3 fatty acids in the average American diet is approximately 20:1, proportionately far more omega-6 fatty acids than in the past. Let's examine these PUFAs and see how they are related to inflammation **(Figure 2).**

Figure 2: Omega-6 and Omega-3 Metabolism in the Body (How They Break Down)

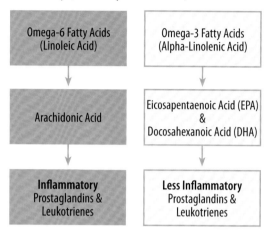

You can see the relationship between omega-6 fatty acids and their highly inflammatory breakdown products and omega-3 fatty acids and their less inflammatory breakdown products. You may be wondering how these inflammatory breakdown products cause harm. One concept to understand is that each cell in our bodies has a cell skin (called a membrane) that is composed, in part, of fatty acids—of both the omega-3 and omega-6 types, as well as others. Fatty acids are readily incorporated into cell membranes, so when it comes to fats, you are indeed what you eat. This means that consuming too much omega-6 and not enough omega-3 fats can alter cell-membrane composition to be more inflammatory. The reason this happens is because omega-6 fatty acids lead to the production of more arachidonic acid (as does saturated fat), which in turn leads to an inflammatory series of events in the body. By contrast, consuming omega-3 fat stimulates the production of eicosapentaenoic acid (EPA) and docosahexaenoic acid (DHA), which generates a series of anti-inflammatory molecules called prostaglandins and leukotrienes.

The good news is that you can make the cells of your body less inflammatory by eating more omega-3s, thereby decreasing your ratio of omega-6s to omega-3s (both in your diet and, consequently, in the cells of your body). Omega-3s have a more beneficial effect on inflammation as they compete for space in the cell membrane with arachidonic acid as well as other inflammatory factors. In order to achieve the optimal 4:1 ratio of omega-6 to omega-3 fatty acids, we have to not only increase our consumption of omega-3 fatty acids, but we must also decrease our consumption of omega-6 fatty acids. Every recipe in this book will help you to do just that.

There is no set recommended daily allowance (RDA) for the intake of omega-3 fatty acids. There is some consensus, however, that an acceptable intake of omega-3s should be between 1 and 2 grams per day and that the omega-6 intake should be no more than four to five times the omega-3 intake. In fact, if you have documented heart disease or high triglyceride levels, the American Heart Association recommends that you eat fish (particularly fatty fish) at least twice a week and consume 2 grams of omega-3 fatty acids (with 1 gram from EPA and 1 gram from DHA) each week.

The next time you go grocery shopping, remember to avoid the following rich sources of omega-6 fatty acids: corn, cottonseed, safflower, sunflower, sesame, and peanut oils; margarine; and prepackaged foods or foods with a long shelf life. Instead, consider incorporating some rich sources of omega-3 fatty acids listed in **Table 3** (see page 12) into your diet.

Table 3: Dietary Sources of Omega-3 Fatty Acids

Food Item	Omega-3 Fatty Acid Content (grams)
Fish/Seafood (4 ounces [114 g])	
Mackerel	2.2
Sardines	1.8
Herring	1.4
Salmon	1.7
Swordfish	1.7
Bluefish	1.7
Cod	0.6
Crab, soft shell	0.6
Scallops	0.5
Tuna (canned in water)	0.3
Lobster	0.1
Nuts/Seeds (1 ounce [28 g])	
Flaxseeds	1.8
Walnuts (14 halves)	2.6
Pecans	0.3
Grains/Beans (½ cup [113 g])	
Soybeans, cooked	0.5
Tofu	0.4
Greens (½ cup [10 g] cooked)	
Spinach	0.1
Kale	0.1
Collard greens	0.1
Oils (1 tablespoon [14 ml])	
Flaxseed	6.9
Canola	1.3
Walnut	1.4
Olive	0.1

Monounsaturated Fats (MUFAs)

Monounsaturated fats are found in particularly high concentrations in olive and canola oils. These types of fats are representative of a Mediterranean-style diet, a dietary pattern that has recently been touted for protective health effects. Monounsaturated fats have proven benefits in preventing heart disease and reducing cholesterol. Olive oil, in particular, may have additional anti-inflammatory powers because of the antioxidant compounds it contains, such as carotenoids and flavonoids. Oleocanthal is a compound rich in olive oil that fights inflammation in a similar fashion to nonsteroidal anti-inflammatory drugs.

Is There a Best Type of Fat?

Most experts would agree that both omega-3 fats and monounsaturated fats are "healthy" types of fats and should therefore be included in our diets. You may be wondering how one type of "healthy" fat stacks up against the others. For that, let's look at **Table 4**.

It is very difficult to make a comparison between these fats because they each have unique features that make them a healthful part of the diet. Let's start by comparing their unsaturated-fat-to-saturated-fat ratio. Canola oil, followed by flax oil, appears to be best in this category. Canola oil also contains less saturated fat and more of the antioxidant vitamin E than olive oil.

Oleic acid is related to oleocanthal, a substance found in newly pressed extra virgin olive oil (which offers the most flavorful and greatest antioxidant benefit). It has a potency similar to nonsteroidal anti-inflammatory drugs. Olive oil is the clear winner in this category. Flax oil is a rich source of omega-3s with the most favorable omega-3 to omega-6 ratio.

Table 4: Comparison of "Healthy" Fats

Fat	Unsaturated/ Saturated Ratio	Oleic Acid (% by weight)	Omega-6 (% by weight)	Omega-3 (% by weight)	Omega-3: Omega-6
Canola Oil	15.7	62	22	10	2:1
Olive Oil	4.6	71	10	1	10:1
Flax Oil	9.0	21	16	53	1:3.5

The point of this illustration is to show that many fats have attractive properties and, like everything else, they should be consumed in moderation as part of an overall healthy diet.

THE BAD FATS
Saturated Fats
Saturated fats have the unsavory reputation of being the original "evil" fats because they have been scientifically shown to increase levels of LDL (bad fats) and decrease levels of HDL (good fats), thus leading to an increased risk of heart disease. Sources of saturated fats in the diet are mainly animal products, including meat, whole-milk dairy products, and egg yolks. Some plant foods are also high in saturated fats, like coconut, palm, and palm kernel oils. Saturated fats of any sources ought to be consumed sparingly. It is recommended that our daily diet contain no more than 10 percent saturated fat.

Trans Fats (TFAs)
It was determined decades ago that saturated fats are harmful and can lead to heart attacks and strokes. Believing that polyunsaturated fats (PUFAs) were healthier than saturated fats, but also knowing that they spoiled more easily, food scientists devised ways to manipulate PUFAs so they were as shelf stable as saturated fats. In order to make it a more stable fat, polyunsaturated fats were heated, causing a change in their shape from *cis* to *trans*; in addition, hydrogen gas was infused into the heated oil, allowing it to partially hydrogenate. As a result, partially hydrogenated vegetable oils (corn, soybean, cottonseed, etc.) were invented that were very shelf stable and could be used in cooking. The problem now is that these supposedly healthier fats—trans-polyunsaturated fats— are also associated with an increased risk of heart attacks and strokes.

Products containing trans fats can often be found in the center aisles of your grocery store. These fats are referred to as the omega-6 fatty acids and, when partially hydrogenated, are even worse because they become trans fats. It should come as no surprise that many baked goods (doughnuts, crackers, cookies) and prepackaged products contain omega-6 fatty acids, especially partially hydrogenated ones (e.g., partially hydrogenated cottonseed oil). Excessive consumption of these types of oils increases our intake of omega-6 fatty acids, which worsens the ratio of omega-6 to omega-3s. Another important consideration is that the way we prepare foods also influences the TFA content of foods. For instance, foods that have been fried in vegetable oils and repeatedly heated will be rich in TFAs. One of the foods likely to contain high amounts of TFAs is french fries from fast food chains that rely on frying in constantly reheated oil.

Because of the clear link between trans fats and heart disease, the Food and Drug Administration now requires that products containing trans fat must identify it on the food label. New York City recently banned use of TFAs in the preparation of restaurant foods. Trans fats are associated with increased cholesterol and markers of inflammation.

WHAT ELSE IN OUR DIETS IS INFLAMMATORY?

Another major nutrition change we have observed in our food industry practices over the last century is an increase in sugar use and consumption. While an optimal ratio of carbs to proteins and fats in our diets is the subject of debate, the negative effect of too much sugar (or simple carbohydrates) in our diets is more clearly understood. Sugar and foods that are made up of simple carbohydrates, also described as high glycemic index foods, are associated with inflammation. The glycemic index is a measure of how much and how rapidly a food's carbohydrate content affects blood-sugar levels after it is eaten. High glycemic index foods include sugared

candies (jelly beans), regular (not diet) soda, and white carbs such as rice, pasta, and bread. Consuming too many of these kinds of foods is associated with high blood-sugar levels and the problem of insulin resistance.

Diets that are low in sugar and simple carbohydrates (low glycemic index) have been shown to be associated with significantly less inflammation than diets that are low fat but high in simple carbohydrates. Diets that are made up of monounsaturated fats, whole grains, lean meats and fish, fruits, and nuts (sometimes termed "Mediterranean style") are associated with less inflammation.

DOES FOOD PREPARATION INFLUENCE INFLAMMATION?

Overcooking food can also increase inflammation. Overcooking or charring foods on the grill can lead to compounds called heat-generated advanced glycation end products (AGEs). These AGEs increase inflammation in the body and have also been shown to increase LDL (bad) cholesterol. To minimize inflammation through food preparation practices, it is best to cook foods by steaming or lightly sautéing.

Figure 3: Food Guide Pyramid Designed to Reduce Dietary Triggers of Inflammation

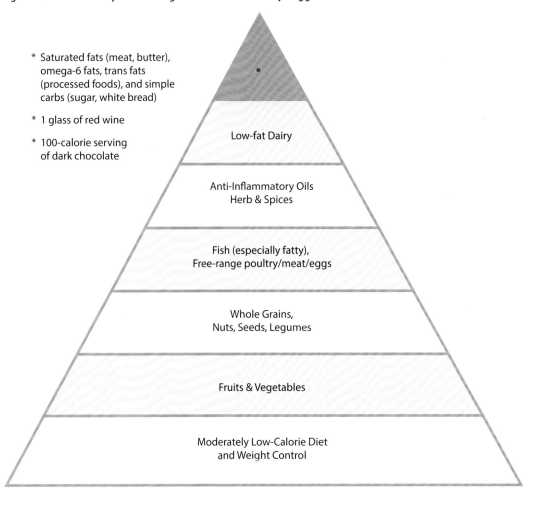

* Saturated fats (meat, butter),
  omega-6 fats, trans fats
  (processed foods), and simple
  carbs (sugar, white bread)

* 1 glass of red wine

* 100-calorie serving
  of dark chocolate

*

Low-fat Dairy

Anti-Inflammatory Oils
Herb & Spices

Fish (especially fatty),
Free-range poultry/meat/eggs

Whole Grains,
Nuts, Seeds, Legumes

Fruits & Vegetables

Moderately Low-Calorie Diet
and Weight Control

FOODS THAT FIGHT INFLAMMATION

Now that we've discussed everything that tends to increase inflammation and that you should try to limit in your diet, let's talk about what you should consider making a more prominent part of your diet. Use the Food Guide Pyramid Designed to Reduce Dietary Triggers of Inflammation (**Figure 3**) as a guide to reducing inflammation through your diet.

Let's start at the bottom of the anti-inflammatory pyramid and work our way to the top.

MODERATELY LOW-CALORIE DIET AND WEIGHT CONTROL

The bottom of the pyramid emphasizes a moderately low-calorie diet and weight control. The rationale for this is that both too much body weight and too many calories have been linked to higher amounts of inflammation.

If you recall, fat tissue releases lots of inflammatory molecules into your bloodstream. The greater amount of fat tissue, especially around the midsection, the more inflammation you are likely to have. To know if you are normal weight or are carrying too many extra pounds, you can calculate your body mass index (BMI) by dividing your body weight in pounds or kilograms (kg) by your height in inches squared or meters squared (m^2). If you are of normal body weight for your height (body mass index [BMI] $\leq$ 25 kg/m^2), then to maintain your weight and to avoid weight gain, you must eat the same number of calories that you burn in a day. There are many websites where you can find out how many calories a person of your age, gender, height, and weight typically burns each day to get a sense of your own daily caloric needs. If you are overweight for your height, then in order to lose weight, you must burn more calories per day than you eat. In order to lose one pound of weight per week, you must either cut back on the daily calories you consume by five hundred calories or burn an additional five hundred calories per day—or the best and most attainable bet is to reduce calories while increasing exercise.

Even if you are of normal weight but consume a very high calorie diet, made up mostly of sugar and fat, you may be introducing inflammation into your body. Sugar, polyunsaturated fat (of the omega-6 type), trans-fatty acids, and saturated fats have all been linked to increased levels of inflammation. So it is smart to minimize sources of these in your diet.

FRUITS AND VEGETABLES

Eating a diet with an abundance of fruits and vegetables is one of the best ways to assure that you are eating in an anti-inflammatory way. Many studies have confirmed the relationship between greater fruit and vegetable consumption and decreased risk of inflammation (lower C-reactive protein) and such oxidative stress-driven diseases as cardiovascular disease and cancer. That's because fruits and vegetables (especially those that are red, orange, or yellow) are a rich source of antioxidants such as carotenoids, vitamin C, and quercetin. Excellent sources of carotenoids include papayas, tangerines, yellow peppers, pumpkins, winter squash, sweet potatoes, carrots, apricots, and cantaloupe. Sources of vitamin C include citrus fruits, tomatoes, berries, peppers, sweet potatoes, broccoli, cauliflower, asparagus, and dark green leafy vegetables. Fruit and vegetable sources of quercetin include berries (blueberries, blackberries, dark cherries), grapefruit, onions, and apples.

There are a few vegetables to be aware of if you are sensitive to food allergies. They are known as "nightshade vegetables" and include eggplant, tomatoes, and potatoes. They contain a chemical called solanine that may trigger an inflammatory response in some people. Other foods that are not vegetables but are often associated with food allergies include eggs, dairy, and wheat products. These foods may also trigger inflammation in some people.

WHOLE GRAINS, NUTS, SEEDS, AND LEGUMES

The beneficial effect of these foods comes in part from the fact that they are high in fiber and are low-glycemic-index foods. These foods have been shown to reduce levels of C-reactive protein, whereas diets high in sugar (refined cereals, sweets, fruit juice, white breads, and pasta) cause rapid increases in blood-sugar levels that trigger the release of insulin and pro-inflammatory chemicals. The key is to avoid highly processed grains and eat organic versions whenever possible. Some individuals may actually have an intolerance to grains containing gluten and will have higher levels of inflammation in response. If you suspect that you might be one of these individuals, it is recommended that you avoid gluten-containing grains.

Table 5: How to Reverse the Damage of Too Much Saturated Fat

Food	Saturated Fat (g)	Total PUFAs (g)	Omega-6 Fat (g)	Omega-3 Fat (g)
Steak (8 ounces [228 g])	13.3	1.232	1.23	0
Salmon (8 ounces [228 g])	2.98	6	3	3

FISH, FREE-RANGE POULTRY/MEAT/EGGS
Eating more cold-water fish is one of the easiest ways to increase your omega-3 fatty acid intake. Mackerel, salmon, and swordfish contain the highest amounts of omega-3s. Despite some recent concern about contaminants found in fish, such as mercury, the health benefits gained from eating them at least twice a week outweigh the risks for most people (exceptions include pregnant women and young children; please consult your health care provider for advice).

What if you are a health-conscious steak lover? Even if you choose to consume steak once in a while, let's see how you can reverse its damage painlessly. Let's work through an example of how to offset the inflammation when you've eaten too many of the omega-6 types of fats. **Table 5** shows the breakdown of fats between steak and salmon.

How can you correct for eating too much of the bad fats? Let's take steak, for instance. If we are trying to attain a 4:1 ratio between omega-6 and omega-3 fatty acids, based on these numbers, we would have to consume only 1 ounce (28 g) of salmon to offset an 8 ounce (228 g) steak. Let's do the math:

8 ounces (228 g) of steak contains 1.2 g of omega-6s

1 ounce (28 g) of salmon contains 0.3 g of omega-3s

Overall ratio of omega-6 to omega-3 = 1.2 : 0.3 = **4:1**

The goal is to cut back on steak and to eat more fish. If you enjoy steak and poultry, choose leaner cuts of free-range meats from animals that have not been corn fed or pumped full of hormones. When purchasing eggs, choose free-range or omega-3 eggs.

ANTI-INFLAMMATORY OILS, HERBS, AND SPICES

Regular consumption of olive, canola, and flax oils is recommended. Each oil is unique in its structure and its properties that influence health, and therefore they should all be included in your diet.

Not only are spices and herbs a great way to add flavor to food, but several of them also contain beneficial anti-inflammatory compounds. Consider adding the following anti-inflammatory spices and herbs to your meals: ginger, rosemary, turmeric, oregano, cayenne, clove, nutmeg, feverfew, and Boswellia.

LOW-FAT DAIRY

Low-fat or nonfat milk, yogurt, and cheese are excellent sources of dairy. They are both a rich source of calcium and are low on the glycemic index. The benefit here is that low-glycemic-index foods do not increase inflammation in the body the way that high glycemic index foods do.

There are a few specific considerations about including dairy products in your diet. The first is that you'll want to purchase dairy foods that are low fat or nonfat because the full-fat versions contain high amounts of inflammatory saturated fats, which offset any benefit of their being low glycemic. Second, be aware that if you are allergic to dairy, eating a dairy product may actually increase inflammation in your body.

SATURATED FATS, OMEGA-6 FATS, TRANS FATS, AND SIMPLE CARBS

Sugar-sweetened soft drinks, refined grains, and processed foods, including meats, have all been associated with elevated markers of inflammation and should be eaten sparingly. Refined grains tend to be low in fiber and have a high glycemic index. When faced with a craving for sweets, consider indulging in antioxidant-rich dark chocolate instead.

Chocolate lovers will be glad to know that dark chocolate is a healthy part of an anti-inflammatory diet (when consumed in moderation, of course). Chocolate has long been touted for its ability to enhance our moods by increasing serotonin levels. Another benefit is that dark chocolate is rich in polyphenols (called catechins) that have antioxidant properties. The highest levels of catechins are found in dark chocolate made from at least 70 percent cocoa. Go for dark chocolate—it contains roughly ten times more catechins and antioxidant activity than does milk chocolate.

ANTI-INFLAMMATORY BEVERAGES

Tea

Similar to dark chocolate, tea contains antioxidant catechins. White, green, and black teas all contain antioxidant catechins to varying degrees. White tea contains the greatest amount, followed by green tea and black tea. The amount of antioxidant content is inversely related to the extent to which the teas have been processed or fermented. White and green teas have been minimally processed and therefore contain the highest level of antioxidants. There are numerous catechins in tea. The primary catechin in white and green tea is epigallocatechin gallate (EGCG). EGCG contains antioxidant properties and stimulates a modest increase in energy expenditure, which may help to enhance weight control.

Many authorities recommend a goal of consuming approximately 300 milligrams of catechins per day, half from EGCG. The exact catechin content of tea is hard to decipher from food labels. A safe bet is to drink at least two to three cups a day.

Wine

Certain properties of wine, especially red wine, seem to have beneficial effects on health when consumed in moderation. It is believed that red wine is responsible for the "French paradox," which refers to the lower rates of heart disease-related deaths observed among the French despite the fact that their diet is high in saturated fat.

Moderate alcohol consumption (one drink per day for women, one to two drinks per day for men) has consistently been linked to lower levels of inflammation, a lower risk of type-2 diabetes, and a lower risk of heart disease. The effect is more profound among red wine drinkers. Like other alcohols, red wine has a thinning effect on blood that makes platelets less sticky and less likely to clot. Red wine, however, outperforms other forms of alcohol because it contains more than 200 health-enhancing antioxidant compounds called polyphenols. The antioxidant activity in a single glass of red wine (a 5-ounce [150 ml] serving) is on average equivalent to twelve glasses of white wine.

One of the most potent polyphenols in red wine is called resveratrol. Resveratrol has received lots of attention lately for its ability to extend life span in animal models. The only other known way to extend life span is by restricting total daily caloric intake by 30 to 40 percent. Resveratrol has been shown to have a broad range of health-enhancing properties, including antioxidant, anti-inflammatory, and antimicrobial capabilities. It has been shown to suppress tumor cells, improve such disease states as cardiovascular disease, cancer, and diabetes, and fight stomach infections such as Helicobacter pylori.

Grape skins and seeds contain the highest level of polyphenols. Because resveratrol is part of the natural defense mechanism of the grape, it increases in response to damp, cool climates, ultraviolet light, and attack by fungal infections. Commonly used pesticides protect wine grapes from infection, but they also decrease their resveratrol content. Therefore, organically grown grapes grown at high altitude in cool, damp climates should contain the greatest content of resveratrol. Pinot noir, Cabernet, and Syrah red wines are most likely to have relatively high resveratrol contents. (Pregnant women or anyone with a history of alcohol abuse should obviously not include wine consumption as an element of their anti-inflammatory diet.)

A New Beginning

Hopefully, you are now convinced that many of the most troubling threats to your health are related to dietary sources of inflammation and that paying attention to food choices and food preparation methods can be of enormous benefit. Remember the following points summarized below as you embark on your anti-inflammatory cooking and eating adventure.

Summary of the Anti-Inflammatory Diet

- Eat calories in moderation by eating smaller portions. Fewer calories means lower body weight, which means less inflammation.

- Avoid "bad" fats (trans fat, saturated fat, too much omega-6 fat) and eat more "good" fats (omega-3 fat, monounsaturated fat).

- Limit your intake of sugar and refined carbohydrates, and eat more high-fiber, low-glycemic-index sources of carbohydrates (i.e., whole grains).

- Enjoy unlimited amounts of antioxidant-rich fruits and vegetables.

- Cook with anti-inflammatory herbs and spices.

- Avoid charred or overgrilled foods.

- Incorporate modest amounts of antioxidant-rich extras such as red wine, dark chocolate, and green tea into your daily diet.

In the chapters that follow, you will find a variety of delicious, simple-to-prepare dishes that can ease your path to reducing dietary sources of inflammation. Here's to an anti-inflammatory lifestyle and better health!

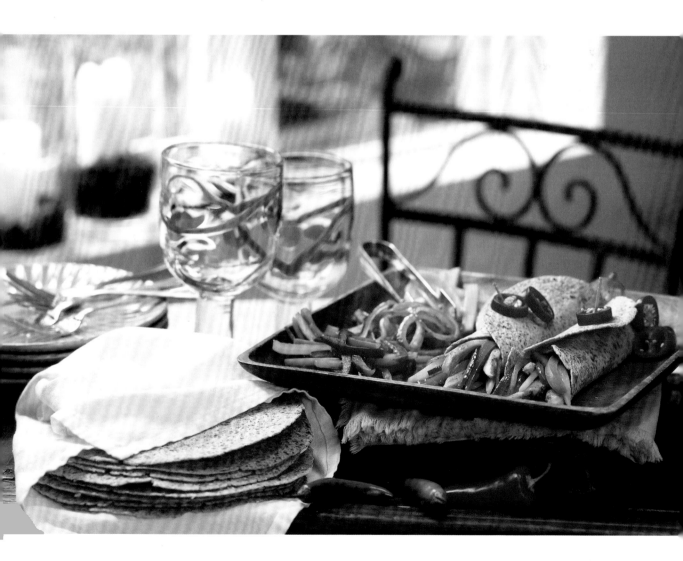

CHAPTER 1

Boost Omega-3s

Adding more unsaturated fats and omega-3 fatty acids to your diet, and reducing saturated and trans fats, is important to developing a healthier way of eating. Unsaturated fats such as flaxseed and canola oil contain important antioxidants to protect your body from oxidative stress and help prevent the development of cancer cells. An adequate source of unsaturated fats assists your body in reducing inflammation and creating more flexible cell membranes, which is important in the prevention of heart disease. Omega-3s have the additional benefit of being a natural blood thinner, which protects against stroke.

Making Changes to Your Diet

If you are making significant changes to your diet, and are on blood pressure medications or anticoagulants to thin the blood, let your physician know about your plan because your medication dose may need to be changed.

Making changes to your diet may seem daunting at first. Most of us are attached to our habits and find it difficult to incorporate new foods into our daily and weekly eating patterns. The best way to build a new diet pattern is make just a few changes at a time into your current pattern, and wait until those changes are well established before making further changes. For example, if you currently eat fish about once a week, plan for a second fish meal in the week. If you do not currently include a soy or other vegetarian main courses in your weekly diet, plan on adding one of these every week.

PLANNING

Planning is an essential tool in your effort to achieve a new eating pattern. By making a plan, you are committing to a goal, and thus are more likely to achieve the change that you desire. Once you have made a plan, make sure that you have the necessary components to carry it out: make shopping lists of ingredients you need, take into account the time and equipment you have available to cook, and consider personal preferences and budget.

EQUIPMENT AND TECHNIQUES

You may also need to purchase new items and equipment for your kitchen, but these investments will definitely pay off as you reap the benefits of healthier eating. For example, an automatic breadmaker is helpful for making breads high in omega-3s (see Chapter 3, "Fabulous Fiber," for recipes). A nut chopper saves time in preparing recipes with nuts, and the resulting pieces will be more uniform.

Using the right cooking techniques, and carefully following recipes, is also a vital part of reshaping your eating pattern. No one is likely to incorporate new dishes into their eating plan if the food is not appealing and delicious!

Buying Fish

With fish, it is important that you buy the freshest available. Gently wash steaks or fillets with cold water and pat with paper towels to dry before starting a recipe. Avoid overcooking fish because it will taste dry and rubbery. When cooking fish, check it often and remove it from the heat source before the fish appears entirely done. It will continue to cook from residual heat for a few minutes, and should be easily flaked with a fork. Serve it as soon as possible to maintain its tender flavor.

You can usually substitute one type of fish for another with similar qualities. For example, recipes calling for salmon often do well with fresh tuna steaks. Cod can be replaced by orange roughy or halibut.

FYI

Trans-fatty acids (TFAs) are bad fats in that they promote inflammation and heart disease. Fortunately, there are a growing number of products in grocery stores that are TFA free, including margarine (which is typically high in TFA). Look for labels stating "non-hydrogenated" or "trans fatty acid free." If the label also states that the product is "light" on calories or contains flaxseed (linseed) oil, all the better!

Polishing Your Oil Techniques

Using good techniques with cooking oil is also important. The flavor of cooking oils, for example, can easily be enhanced by the addition of a few simple ingredients. To add a citrus flavor, add lemon or orange zest to the oil, allowing it to absorb the flavor for eight to ten minutes before using it in the recipe. For savory dishes, add one to two minced garlic cloves, a tablespoon (15 g) of Dijon mustard, or two to three tablespoons (7.5 to 11 g) of minced fresh cilantro. When preparing oil to pan fry fish, use just enough oil to coat the bottom of the pan in a thin layer, and wait until it is very hot before adding the fish. This will give the fish a nice golden crust.

Polyunsaturated oils break down with repeated exposure to heat, light, and oxygen, so it is important to use fresh oil every time you cook, and to keep your oils stored in the refrigerator or in a cool, dark place with the lid tightly closed. Avoid using flaxseed or walnut oil with stove-top cooking because they are oxidized by heat. Use these oils for salad dressings and cold dishes instead.

Presenting Your Dishes

Attractive presentation of your dishes is essential when serving foods at home. Take an extra five minutes to prepare a garnish that will highlight one or more of the ingredients in the dish. Prepare foods with a variety of contrasting colors for eye appeal. Arrange the food items on a serving dish or individual plates in a pleasing design. You'll be surprised at the difference presentation can make in giving your dishes a gourmet look!

FYI
Eggs vary in content according to how the hens are kept and what they are fed. Eggs from free-range hens are likely to have a healthier fat profile than those from caged hens. They tend to be lower in saturated fat and higher in omega-3s. The best eggs to purchase are free-range eggs advertised to be high in omega-3s.

Omega-3 Super Ingredients

The omega-3 fatty-acid content of these recipes can be boosted by purchasing the right products in your local grocery store. With so much positive information coming out about the benefits of omega-3s, manufacturers are modifying their products to provide a richer omega-3 content. Here are some examples:

EGGS
Hens fed special vegetarian diets lay eggs that are higher in omega-3 content. Many producers are following the trend and feeding their hens healthier diets. While these eggs are definitely "a cut above" the rest, you'll still want to be moderate in using eggs in your diet, especially if you are trying to reduce your blood cholesterol.

OIL
Look for blended oils made from canola, soy, and olive oil, and margarine made from these oils. These products are an excellent source of omega-3 fatty acids and are very versatile in the kitchen. Blending the oils makes them more stable for cooking. Olive oil is a beneficial component in the blend not so much for its omega-3 content, but because it does not break down easily when subjected to higher heat. Walnut oil is also high in omega-3s and lends a delicious flavor to cold food recipes.

FLAXSEED

Flaxseed can be bought in many major grocery stores. Look for it in the natural foods section. It is an excellent source of omega-3 fatty acids and adds a nutty flavor to pancakes and baked goods. Whole flaxseeds are easily ground into a powder by using an electric coffee bean grinder. (Just make sure to rinse the coffee residue out before grinding the flaxseed.) Grind just enough for use in your recipe because the flaxseed oil begins to break down once the protective shell has been fractured. If you have leftover ground flaxseed, it can be stored for a short time (less than thirty days) in the refrigerator in an opaque container. Ground flaxseed can also be used to replace eggs or oil in a recipe. To use it as an egg substitute, mix one tablespoon of ground flaxseed with three tablespoons of water and whisk until the mixture is frothy. This mixture is the equivalent of one egg.

FISH

Most Americans do not eat the recommended number of servings of fish each week, and recent statistics indicate that 99 percent of people in the United States do not consume enough omega-3 fatty acids. One reason for this low consumption may be concern over mercury levels in fish; however, studies on this topic show that the benefits of fish consumption far outweigh any potential risks.

Although fatty fish such as mackerel and salmon offer the highest amounts of omega-3s, other fish such as tilapia and butterfish can be combined with other ingredients to boost the omega-3 content in dishes that are both healthful and delicious!

FYI
Pregnant women should make sure to get DHA in their diets because it is critical for fetal brain, eye, and vascular system development. This is especially important during the last trimester. The American Heart Association confirms that the benefits of eating fish twice per week for pregnant and lactating women, as well as children, outweigh potential risks related to mercury intake. It recommends, however, that these two groups avoid eating shark, swordfish, king mackerel, and tilefish.

Grilled Fish Tacos with Mango

Fish tacos are a popular item along the western coast of Mexico, where many varieties are served at local restaurants. This version is not only tasty, but it is also full of antioxidants and omega-3s. Any firm white fish fillet, such as cod, can be substituted for the mahimahi.

---

1 pound (455 g) mahimahi fillets

2 tablespoons (28 ml) canola oil

2 tablespoons (28 mg) omega-3-rich margarine, melted

Juice of 1 lime

1½ teaspoons salt, divided

1 teaspoon chili powder

½ teaspoon crushed red pepper

½ teaspoon garlic powder

¼ teaspoon oregano

½ teaspoon ground cumin

3 mangoes

¼ cup (15 g) cilantro, chopped

8 whole-wheat flour tortillas

Soak fish fillets in cold water 1 to 2 minutes. Pat dry with a paper towel and place in a shallow dish. In a medium-size bowl, whisk together the canola oil, margarine, lime juice, 1 teaspoon of salt, and the remaining dried spices. Pour mixture over the fish. Cover and marinate 30 to 45 minutes in the refrigerator.

Meanwhile, peel mangoes and cut into ½-inch (1-cm) cubes. Mix with cilantro and remaining salt.

Preheat grill to medium-high. Remove fish from the marinade, place on the grill, and cook 2 to 3 minutes on each side, depending on the thickness of the fillets. Fish should flake easily with a fork.

Place tortillas on the grill and grill 10 to 15 seconds on each side. Fill with fish fillets and mango topping.

Yield: 8 servings

Nutritional Analysis: *Each serving provides 240 calories; 7 g fat; 17 g protein; 31 g net carbohydrate; 3 g dietary fiber; and 53 mg cholesterol.*

Tangy Scallop Salad

Scallops are a good source of vitamin B12, a nutrient that is important to cardiovascular health. Just 4 ounces of scallops contain over a third of the recommended daily value of this vitamin. Because scallops are highly perishable, they are immediately shelled, washed, and frozen, or packed in ice, after being harvested. Fresh scallops should be white and firm, without any browning. Frozen scallops should be solid, without frost in the packing.

---

2 tablespoons (28 ml) extra virgin olive oil

2 tablespoons (18 g) seafood seasoning

1 pound (455 g) scallops

4 corn cobs, cooked

1 yellow bell pepper, seeded and diced

1 red bell pepper, seeded and diced

2 mangoes, peeled and diced

1 avocado, peeled and diced

3 tablespoons (40 ml) lemon juice

3 tablespoons (40 ml) lime juice

5 cups (100 g) mixed greens

3 tablespoons (12 g) cilantro, chopped

1 lime, cut into wedges

Heat a medium-size skillet over medium-high heat and add the olive oil. Place scallops in a bowl and season with seafood seasoning. When the oil is hot, add the scallops and sauté until they turn opaque, 3 to 4 minutes. Remove from heat and set aside. Remove the kernels from the corn cobs.

In a large mixing bowl, combine corn kernels, bell peppers, mangoes, avocado, and lemon and lime juices. Toss well. Add the scallops and toss gently until well mixed.

Divide the mixed greens among 4 individual serving plates. Top with the scallop salad, sprinkle with cilantro, and garnish with a lime wedge.

Yield: 4 servings

Nutritional Analysis: Each serving provides 525 calories; 19 g fat; 44 g protein; 44 g net carbohydrate; 11 g dietary fiber; and 81 mg cholesterol.

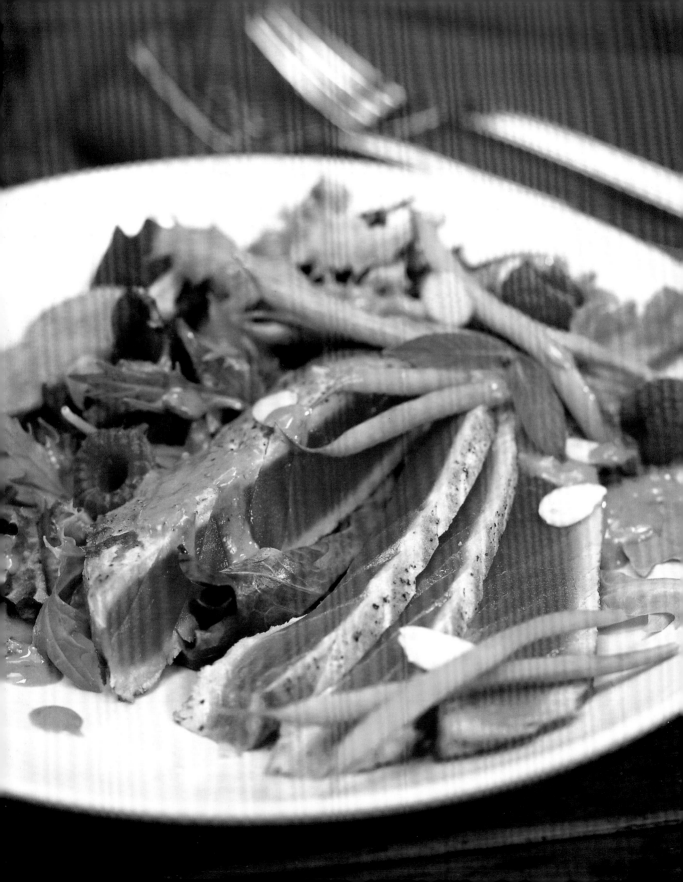

Tuna Steak Salad
with Fresh Raspberry Walnut Dressing

Making your own salad dressing is simple, but if you wish to substitute a favorite commercial dressing, this salad will still be delicious.

For the dressing:

1 pint (300 g) fresh raspberries

½ cup (60 g) walnuts

1 tablespoon (1.5 g) sugar substitute

2 tablespoons (28 ml) raspberry or apple cider vinegar

1 tablespoon (14 ml) lemon juice

2 tablespoons (28 ml) walnut oil

1 tablespoon (15 g) Dijon mustard

1 tablespoon (6 g) fresh mint leaves, finely chopped

⅛ teaspoon black pepper

For the salad:

Four 5-ounce (140 g) fresh tuna steaks

Canola oil spray

Salt and pepper to taste

1 pound (455 g) mixed baby greens

8 ounces (225 g) fresh slender green beans, trimmed

½ cup (60 g) slivered almonds

1 fresh lemon, cut into 4 wedges

Combine dressing ingredients in a blender and blend until smooth. Place in refrigerator to chill.

Spray tuna steaks lightly with canola oil on both sides. Season with salt and pepper to taste. Place tuna on grill and cook 4 to 5 minutes on each side, turning only once. Steam green beans until crisp tender and rinse with cold water.

Rinse mixed baby greens and divide among 4 dinner plates. Arrange green beans, tuna, and almonds on top of mixed greens. Place a lemon wedge on each plate. Serve with dressing.

Yield: 4 servings

Nutritional Analysis: Each serving provides 560 calories; 33 g fat; 50 g protein; 10 g net carbohydrate; 11 g dietary fiber; and 69 mg cholesterol.

Citrus Pan-Seared Tuna Steaks with Fresh Salsa

Tuna tastes best and is most tender when not overcooked. Cook the
tuna steaks for a short time over high heat, searing the edges while
the middle remains rare. Once it is cooked to about ¼-inch (6-mm) deep
(check between the flakes for doneness), remove from the pan.
This dish goes especially well with Mango Pecan Rice (page 73).

For the salsa:

2 tomatoes, peeled, seeds removed, and
chopped

1 clove garlic, minced

3 tablespoons (12 g) fresh cilantro,
chopped

1 tablespoon (14 ml) lime juice

1 jalapeno or other hot pepper, seeded
and minced, optional

Salt and pepper to taste

For the tuna steaks:

Eight 4-ounce (115 g) boneless tuna steaks

2 cups (475 ml) orange juice

3 cloves fresh garlic, finely minced

Sea salt

Black pepper

2 tablespoons (28 ml) olive oil, divided

4 bell peppers: 1 red, 1 green, 1 yellow,
1 orange, thinly sliced

2 red onions, thinly sliced

To make the salsa: Combine the tomatoes, garlic, cilantro, lime juice, and jalapeno pepper in a medium-size bowl. Season with salt and pepper, and set aside.

To prepare the tuna steaks: Place tuna steaks in a baking dish. Mix orange juice with minced garlic, pour over steaks, and marinate for 15 minutes. Drain off orange juice mix and season tuna steaks to taste with sea salt and pepper. Heat a skillet over medium-high heat and add 1 tablespoon (14 ml) olive oil. When oil is hot, place tuna in pan and cook until the bottom is light brown. Flip the steaks, and cook until browned on the other side (about 45 to 60 seconds each side). The center will still be slightly red. Set steaks on a serving dish, cover with aluminum foil, and set in a warm place.

Add the remaining olive oil to skillet and sauté the bell peppers and onions until soft. Serve over tuna steaks, with fresh salsa on the side.

Yield: 8 servings

*Nutritional Analysis: Each serving provides 300 calories; 11 g fat; 36 g protein;
13 g net carbohydrate; 2 g dietary fiber; and 56 mg cholesterol.*

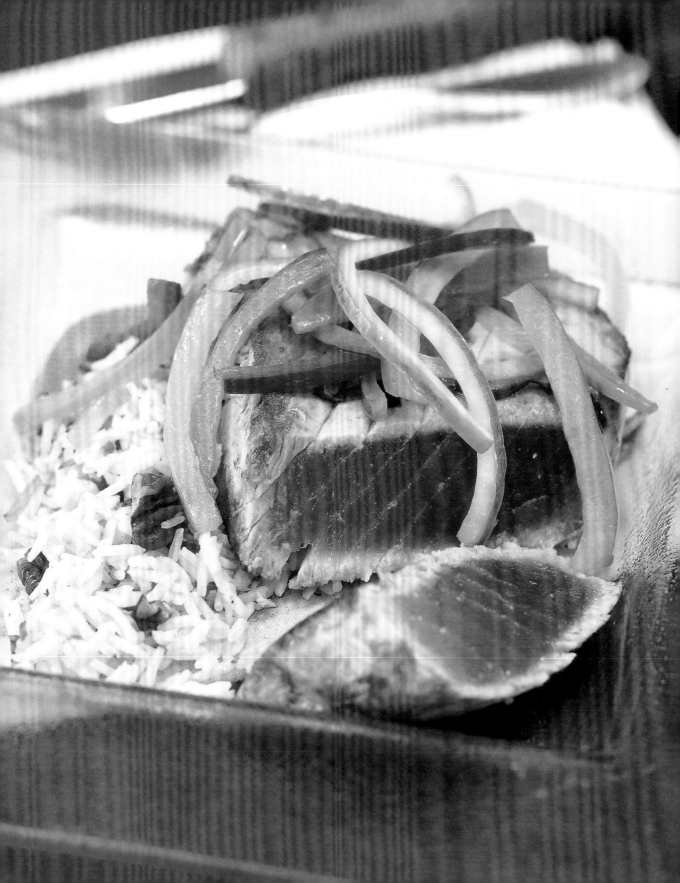

Curried Fish over Basmati Rice

Tilapia and red snapper are good choices for this recipe, but any
white fish fillet will work well. For more fiber, and a nuttier flavor,
substitute brown rice for basmati, and allow it to simmer for
35 to 40 minutes, using the same amount of water.

1½ cups (275 g) basmati rice

2 tablespoons (28 ml) canola oil

1 yellow onion, finely sliced

1 tablespoon (8 g) curry powder

½ teaspoon ground cumin

½ teaspoon ground coriander

¼ teaspoon turmeric

½ teaspoon cayenne pepper, optional

1 bell pepper, cored and thinly sliced

Four 5-ounce (140 g) fish fillets

2 large tomatoes, diced

¼ cup (60 ml) hot water

Place rice in a large sauce pan, and add 3 cups (950 ml) water. Bring to a boil, reduce heat, and simmer 18 to 20 minutes, or until all of the liquid is absorbed.

In a large skillet, heat canola oil over medium-high heat. Add onions and sauté 1 to 2 minutes. Add spices and bell pepper, and cook 1 to 2 minutes longer, stirring constantly. Place fish fillets in the pan and spoon spice mixture over the top. Add tomatoes and water to the dish. Once the liquid comes to a boil, turn heat to medium, cover, and cook 8 to 10 minutes or until fish turns opaque and flakes easily with a fork.

Serve over rice.

Yield: 4 servings

Nutritional Analysis: Each serving provides 520 calories;
8 g fat; 38 g protein; 73 g net carbohydrate;
4 g dietary fiber; and 78 mg cholesterol.

FYI

There are several types of omega-3s. Fish contain the omega-3s docosahexaenoic acid (DHA) and eicosapentaenoic acid (EPA). Vegetable oils such as canola, soybean, and flaxseed/linseed, as well as walnuts, contain alpha-linolenic acid (ALA). Scientific evidence indicates that DHA and EPA significantly reduce blood triglyceride levels. Alpha-linolenic acid also is beneficial, but not as much as fish oil omega-3s. The human body can convert ALA to EPA and DHA, but this conversion is minimal.

[handwritten note: Mar. 29/22 Very good Used Haddock Not too hot/spicy]

Herbed Rockfish

Rockfish is also called Pacific snapper. If you can't find fresh rockfish, trout will do just as well. The garnish is an important factor in the anti-inflammatory character of this dish because tomatoes are rich in cancer-fighting lycopene, and both tomatoes and lemons are a good source of the antioxidant vitamin C.

1½ pounds (680 g) fresh rockfish fillets

2 egg whites

1½ (20 ml) tablespoons nonfat milk

1⅓ (19 ml) tablespoons canola oil

1 cup (245 g) nonfat plain yogurt

1 tablespoon (14 ml) lemon juice

1 tablespoon (4 g) oregano

1 tablespoon (4 g) fresh parsley, finely chopped

1 tablespoon (7.5 g) pimento, finely minced

1 teaspoon garlic, finely minced

1 teaspoon ground black pepper

1 teaspoon thyme

6 slices whole-wheat bread, toasted

¼ cup (30 g) flaxseed, ground

¼ cup (60 ml) extra virgin olive oil

1 pint (350 g) cherry tomatoes, halved

2 fresh lemons, cut into wedges

Rinse rockfish fillets in cold water, remove skin, and check for bones. Pat dry with paper towels. In a medium-size mixing bowl, whisk together egg whites, nonfat milk, canola oil, yogurt, and lemon juice. Place in a pie pan or shallow dish. Place the next 8 ingredients (oregano through flaxseed) in a food processor and process until finely ground. Place in a separate shallow dish.

Heat olive oil in a large skillet. Dredge each fillet in the spice mixture first, followed by the yogurt blend, and then again in the spice mixture, pressing the crumbs lightly into the fish for the final coating. Place fillets in hot oil. When the underside begins to brown, turn fillets over, and reduce heat to medium-low. Cook an additional 15 to 20 minutes, or until fish flakes easily.

Serve with cherry tomatoes and lemon wedges.

Yield: 8 servings

Nutritional Analysis: Each serving provides 280 calories; 14 g fat; 26 g protein; 12 g net carbohydrate; 3 g dietary fiber; and 38 mg cholesterol.

Italian-Style Halibut over Croutons

Kalamata olives are named for Kalamata, Greece, where they originated. They can be cured in a number of different ways. Dry-cured kalamatas are packed in salt and rubbed with olive oil. Kalamatas are also sold packed in vinegar. Fresh, unprocessed olives are inedible because they are extremely bitter.

---

4 tablespoons (56 ml) extra virgin olive oil

2 teaspoons garlic, finely chopped, divided

2 tablespoons (8 g) fresh basil, finely chopped

1 small baguette

Olive oil spray

Four 6-ounce (170 g) halibut fillets

Salt and pepper to taste

½ teaspoon crushed red pepper, optional

1 pint (350 g) grape tomatoes

½ cup (50 g) pitted kalamata olives

1½ tablespoons (13 g) capers

4 anchovies, chopped, optional

½ cup (75 g) chopped tomatoes

¼ cup (15 g) parsley, finely chopped

Whisk together the olive oil, 1 teaspoon of the garlic, and basil. Let stand for 15 minutes to allow the oil to absorb the flavor. To prepare the croutons, slice the baguette into ½-inch (1-cm) slices, and spray both sides with olive oil spray. Toast under the broiler until golden brown. Set aside.

Lightly brush the halibut fillets with the olive oil blend, and season with salt, pepper, and red pepper (if desired). Arrange the halibut on a grill or under a broiler, and cook, turning once, until it flakes easily with a fork, about 3 minutes per side.

Meanwhile, spray a sauté pan lightly with olive oil and sauté the grape tomatoes, olives, capers, and anchovies (if desired) 4 to 5 minutes, stirring often. Add chopped tomatoes and remaining garlic and cook an additional 3 to 4 minutes. Add halibut fillets and gently spoon sauce over fillets until well coated.

Place 2 or 3 croutons on each plate, and top with a halibut fillet and enough sauce to decoratively cover the rounds. Sprinkle with fresh parsley.

Yield: 4 servings

Nutritional Analysis: Each serving provides 460 calories; 24 g fat; 49 g protein; 10 g net carbohydrate; 2 g dietary fiber; and 73 mg cholesterol.

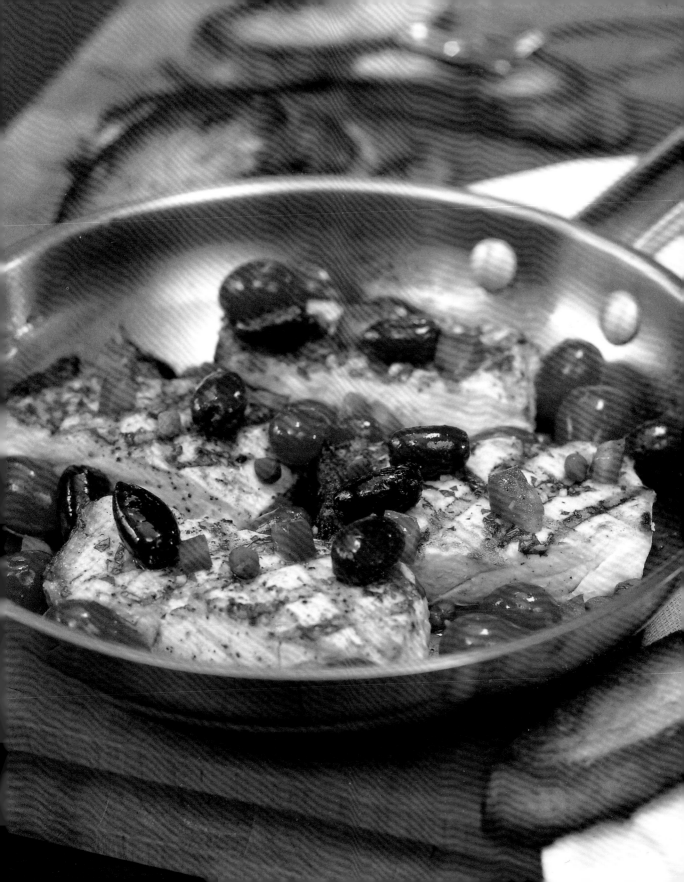

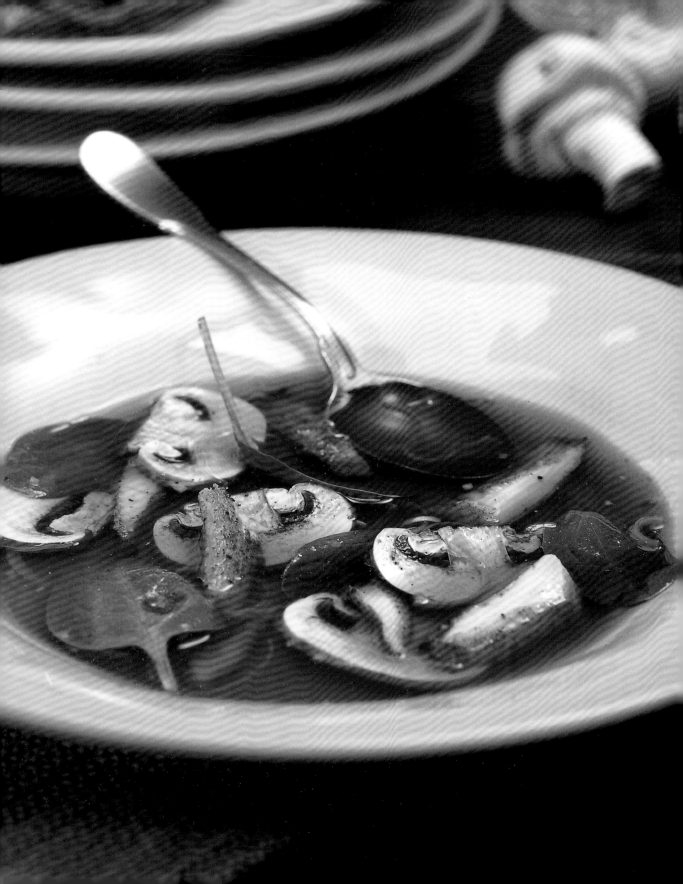

Leek and Spinach Soup with Tilapia

Tilapia is an excellent fish to use in this dish, although lake trout is very tasty as well. For the vegetarian palate, substitute firm tofu. The spinach in the soup is beneficial as it contains at least thirteen different flavonoid compounds that function as antioxidants. Spinach is also very high in vitamin K.

---

6 cups (1.5 L) vegetable
  or 98 percent fat-free chicken broth
2 cups (200 g) mushrooms, sliced
2 leeks, thinly sliced
½ teaspoon garlic, minced

Canola oil spray
6 ounces (168 g) tilapia fillets
  (or firm tofu, cubed)
1 tablespoon (9 g) seafood seasoning
2 cups (40 g) fresh spinach leaves

Bring broth to a boil and add mushrooms, leeks, and garlic. Reduce heat and allow the soup to simmer 15 minutes. Meanwhile, spray a frying pan with canola oil and place over medium-high heat. Sprinkle the fish fillets (or tofu) with the seafood seasoning, and sear in the pan 2 to 3 minutes on each side. Remove from heat, add to the soup, and simmer an additional 5 minutes. Two to 3 minutes prior to serving, add the fresh spinach leaves and allow to soften and wilt.

Yield: 4 servings

Nutritional Analysis: Each serving provides 140 calories; 3 g fat; 17 g protein; 8 g net carbohydrate; 3 g dietary fiber; and 38 mg cholesterol.

FYI

The American Heart Association recommends eating fish at least two times per week—especially such fatty fish as salmon, mackerel, lake trout, herring, sardines, and albacore tuna—due to their high omega-3 content. People with coronary heart disease are advised to consume about 1 gram of EPA and DHA per day, preferably from oily fish. People who have elevated triglycerides might need 2 to 4 grams of EPA and DHA per day. Fish oil supplements should not be consumed without consulting a physician.

Nutty Granola

Granola is a great way to get your fiber in the morning, and it's a cinch to make at home. This recipe has plenty of nuts to boost the omega-3 content. Granola will stay freshest if stored in an airtight container in the refrigerator.

½ cup water

¼ cup (55 g) brown sugar

½ cup (170 g) honey

¾ cup (165 g) omega-3-rich margarine, melted

1 teaspoon vanilla extract

7 cups (525 g) rolled oats

½ cup (60 g) flaxseed, ground

1 cup (70 g) unsweetened coconut, flaked

½ cup (112 g) sunflower seeds

1 cup (125 g) walnuts, finely chopped

½ cup (62 g) almonds, slivered

½ cup (62 g) pecans, finely chopped

½ teaspoon salt

1 cup (175 g) dried apricots, chopped

½ cup (75 g) dates or prunes, chopped

1 cup (112 g) wheat germ

Preheat oven to 350°F (180°C, or gas mark 4).

In a sauce pan, bring the water to a boil, reduce heat, and add the brown sugar, honey, and margarine. Once the sugar dissolves, remove the mixture from the heat and add vanilla extract. In a large bowl, mix together the oats, flaxseed, coconut, sunflower seeds, walnuts, almonds, pecans, and salt. Pour the honey mixture over the oat mixture, and stir well to coat all of the ingredients.

Line a 9 × 13-inch (22.5 × 32.5-cm) baking pan with parchment paper and cover evenly with the granola mixture. Bake 15 to 20 minutes on the middle rack of the oven, stirring often. Set aside to cool.

Once the mixture is cool, stir in the dried fruit and wheat germ and enjoy!

Yield: 28 servings, about ½ cup each

Nutritional Analysis: Each serving provides 280 calories; 16 g fat; 8 g protein; 25 g net carbohydrate; 5 g dietary fiber; and 0 mg cholesterol.

Pecan-Encrusted Salmon Fillets

This delicious salmon recipe will make a fish lover out of anyone. For best results, chop the pecans in a blender until the consistency resembles cornmeal. Keeping the skin on during cooking will ensure a high omega-3 fatty-acid content, and will deliver the richest flavor. Once the fish is ready to serve, you can remove the skin, or serve as is.

2-pound (455 g) salmon fillet, with skin

2 egg whites

1½ (20 ml) tablespoons nonfat milk

1⅓ (19 ml) tablespoons canola oil

1½ cups (88 g) pecans, finely crushed

½ teaspoon celery seed, ground

¼ teaspoon dried mustard

¼ teaspoon crushed red pepper

¼ teaspoon black pepper

⅛ teaspoon bay leaves, ground

⅛ teaspoon allspice

⅛ teaspoon paprika

½ teaspoon salt

1 orange, sliced

4 tablespoons (56 ml) orange juice

4 to 8 fresh parsley sprigs

Preheat oven to 350°F (180°C, or gas mark 4). Place oven rack in the middle position.

Rinse the salmon in cold water, and pat dry with paper towels. Cut into 8 portions. Whisk egg whites, nonfat milk, and canola oil together in a bowl, and place in a shallow dish. Mix pecans, spices, and salt, and place in a separate shallow dish, spreading evenly over the bottom. Dredge each salmon fillet, top side only, in the egg-white mixture first, followed by the pecan mixture, pressing down so pecans adhere. Repeat this process if you prefer a thicker pecan crust.

Place salmon fillets on a broiler pan, skin side down. Bake for approximately 15 minutes, or until salmon is nearly cooked through. Top each fillet with 1 or 2 orange slices and a tablespoon (14 ml) of orange juice. Bake an additional 3 to 4 minutes. Salmon should be opaque all the way through and flake easily with a fork. Serve immediately with orange garnishes and parsley.

Yield: 8 servings

Nutritional Analysis: Each serving provides 450 calories; 32 g fat; 36 g protein; 3 g net carbohydrate; 3 g dietary fiber; and 88 mg cholesterol.

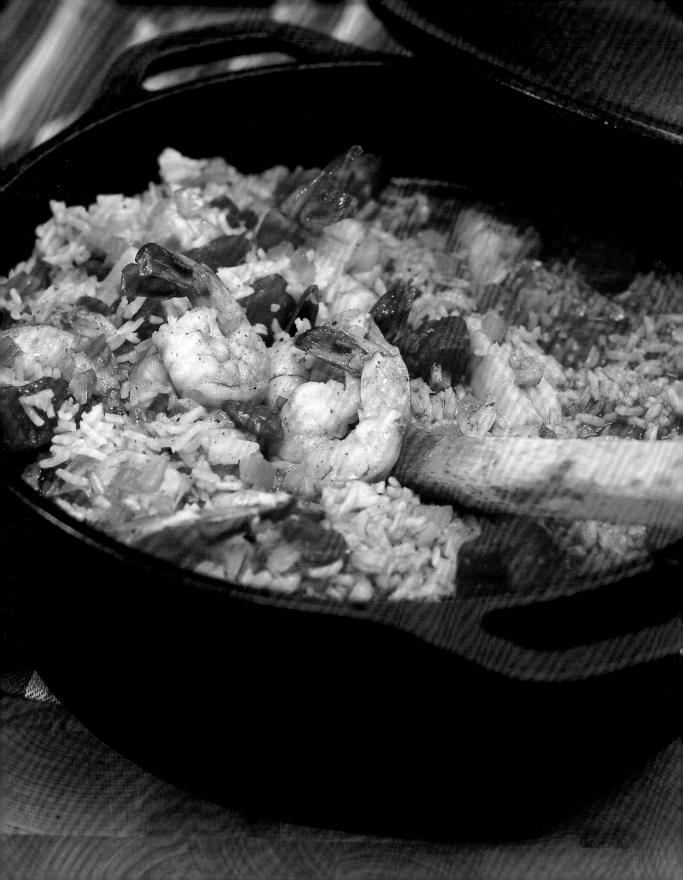

Seafood Jambalaya

In addition to providing omega-3 fatty acids, scallops are also a good source of magnesium and potassium, which are beneficial to the cardiovascular system. Four ounces (115 g) of scallops provide almost 15 percent of the average recommended daily value for omega-3s.

---

2 tablespoons (28 ml) canola oil

1 red onion, finely chopped

3 celery stalks, finely chopped

1 medium green bell pepper, diced

1½ teaspoons garlic, finely chopped

½ teaspoon salt

¼ teaspoon black pepper, ground

2 pounds (1 kg) fresh white fish fillets, cut into large pieces

3 cups (705 ml) vegetable broth

2 cups (370 g) long-grain rice

Two 10-ounce (280 g) cans diced tomatoes

1 teaspoon hot pepper sauce

1 pound (455 g) medium-size raw shrimp, peeled and deveined

½ pound (225 g) fresh scallops

Heat canola oil in a large skillet over medium-high heat. Sauté onion, celery, bell pepper, and garlic 1 to 2 minutes, stirring. Add salt, pepper, and fish fillets, and sauté for another 2 to 3 minutes, turning the fillets over midway through. Add vegetable broth, rice, diced tomatoes, and hot pepper sauce, and bring to a boil. Reduce heat and let simmer for 15 minutes. Stir in shrimp and scallops and cook, covered, 10 minutes longer, until rice is tender and broth has been absorbed.

Yield: 8 servings

Nutritional Analysis: Each serving provides 480 calories; 12 g fat; 44 g protein; 43 g net carbohydrate; 3 g dietary fiber; and 190 mg cholesterol.

Smoked Salmon
on Cucumber Rounds

Party appetizers can be healthful as well as delicious. These cucumber rounds
will disappear quickly, providing valuable omega-3s and fiber for your guests.
Make sure the cucumbers have been refrigerated long enough to be cool tasting.

---

8 ounces (225 g) light cream cheese,
softened

2 tablespoons (28 ml) fat-free
half-and-half

¼ cup (15 g) parsley, finely chopped

½ pound (225 g) smoked salmon,
finely chopped

1 teaspoon lemon zest

¼ cup (58 g) low-fat sour cream

2 English cucumbers

In a medium-size mixing bowl, mix together all ingredients except the cucumbers. Blend well.
Place in refrigerator for 1 to 2 hours to chill. Peel and slice the cucumbers, and place rounds on a
paper towel to slightly dry one side.

Arrange cucumber rounds on a serving plate. Place a small amount of salmon mixture on the
dry side of each cucumber round (about ½ teaspoon).

Yield: About 40 pieces (10 servings of 4 rounds each)

*Nutritional Analysis: Each serving provides 110 calories; 6 g fat;
8 g protein; 5 g net carbohydrate; 1 g dietary fiber;
and 19 mg cholesterol.*

FYI
Many commercial
food companies add
omega-3s to their products,
but they typically do not
specify which type of omega-3
fatty acids have been added.
Unless specified, the most
common omega-3 additive
is alpha-linolenic acid
(ALA).

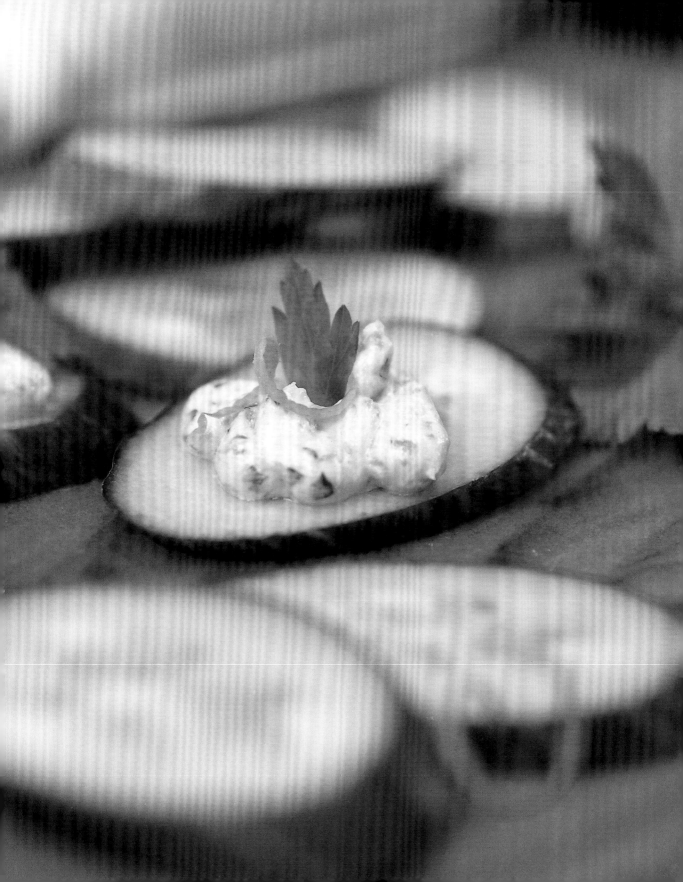

Smoked Salmon Sushi

In addition to its high omega-3 content, salmon is an excellent source of vitamins D, B12, and niacin (B3), and the trace mineral selenium. Several studies have proven that a diet rich in omega-3s offers significant protection against macular degeneration.

1¼ cups (295 ml) water

1 cup (195 g) sushi rice

1½ tablespoons (20 ml) rice vinegar

1½ teaspoons sugar

1 teaspoon salt

4 ounces (115 g) smoked salmon

4 nori seaweed sheets
  (about 7¼" × 8" [18 × 20 cm])

Accompaniments: low-sodium soy sauce
  and wasabi paste, optional

Using a cooking pot with a tight-fitting lid, bring water to a boil on high heat. Add rice, cover, and reduce heat. Simmer 18 to 20 minutes, turn off heat, and allow the rice to stand for 10 minutes. Place rice in a large mixing bowl and sprinkle with vinegar, sugar, and salt. Mix with a wooden spoon, and allow rice to cool.

Slice smoked salmon into strips, about ½-inch (1-cm) wide. Prepare each sushi roll as follows: Place 1 seaweed sheet on a clean, dry surface or bamboo mat, shiny side down, with the longer side across the top and bottom. Place ½ cup (83 g) cooked rice onto the seaweed, and carefully spread evenly over the sheet, leaving 1 inch (2.5 cm) exposed at the right edge. Place strips of salmon (about 1 ounce [28 g]) in a straight line in the middle of the rice, parallel to the exposed edge.

Carefully roll so as not to tear the seaweed, starting at the left edge, ending just before the right edge. Tuck rice in at the edges of the roll. Run a wet finger along the exposed edge of the seaweed, and complete rolling, pressing down to seal the edge to the roll. Slice into pieces ¾-inch (2-cm) wide, using a sharp, slightly wet knife.

Serve with low-sodium soy sauce and Japanese horseradish (wasabi) if desired.

Yield: About 28 pieces of sushi (4 servings of 7 pieces each)

Nutritional Analysis: Each serving provides 110 calories; 4 g fat; 7 g protein; 12 g net carbohydrate; 0 g dietary fiber; and 18 mg cholesterol.

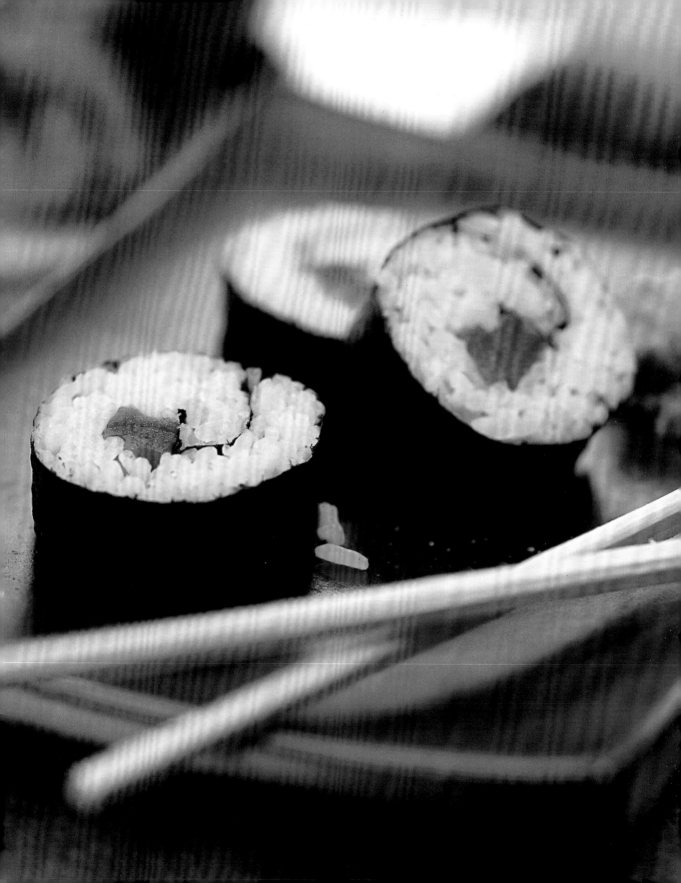

South American Fish Stew with Quinoa

Quinoa is an excellent food for vegetarians because it is rich in
protein and is considered a complete protein, which means that
it contains all of the essential amino acids. Quinoa is high in
iron, potassium, riboflavin, magnesium, zinc, copper, and folate.
It is cooked much like rice and has a delicious, nutty flavor.

One 14½-ounce (405 g) can of diced
  tomatoes

1 bunch scallions, finely sliced

Juice of half a lime

¼ cup (15 g) cilantro, finely chopped

1½ pounds (680 g) red snapper

½ pound (225 g) fresh shrimp, peeled
  and deveined

¾ cup (145 g) quinoa

1½ cups (355 ml) water or 98 percent
  fat-free chicken broth

½ cup (120 ml) coconut milk

Sprigs of fresh cilantro

In a large bowl, mix together the tomatoes, scallions, lime juice, and cilantro. Place the fish and shrimp in a shallow dish and pour tomato mixture over. Cover and refrigerate overnight.

Place quinoa and water (or broth) in a large saucepan. Bring to a boil, turn down heat, cover, and simmer 20 to 30 minutes, or until the grains are soft and the water is completely absorbed. Remove from heat and set aside.

Place the fish, shrimp, and tomato marinade in a large skillet. Heat over medium-high heat until liquid reaches a boil. Reduce heat and simmer for 20 minutes. Add quinoa and coconut milk and cook 5 to 8 minutes longer.

Serve garnished with fresh cilantro sprigs.

Yield: 4 servings

Nutritional Analysis: *Each serving provides 430 calories; 11 g fat; 53 g protein; 25 g net carbohydrate; 5 g dietary fiber; and 174 mg cholesterol.*

Spicy Herb-Encrusted Catfish

This recipe is adapted from a popular dish found on the
Eastern shore of Maryland. It's great with red potatoes or in a sandwich.
Double the crushed red pepper, if you dare!

For the spice mixture:

¼ cup (20 g) coriander seeds

1½ teaspoons cumin seeds

2 teaspoons seafood seasoning

½ tablespoon crushed red pepper

½ teaspoon ground cardamom

1 tablespoon (12 g) raw sugar

1 tablespoon (18 g) kosher salt

1 teaspoon fresh ground black pepper

Four 6-ounce (170 g) catfish fillets

½ cup (60 g) flaxseed, ground

Canola oil spray

For the garnish:

Several large sprigs of fresh cilantro

1 medium-size tomato, quartered

1 lemon, quartered

Preheat oven to 350°F (180°C, or gas mark 4). Place the spice mixture ingredients into a medium-size mixing bowl, and blend well. Put the mixture into a pie pan. Wash catfish fillets and pat dry with paper towels. Place ground flaxseed into a separate pie pan. Alternately dredge fillets in spice mixture and flaxseed. Spray baking sheet with canola oil spray. Place fillets on baking sheet and bake 15 to 18 minutes, or until center portion of fish flakes easily with a fork. Broil pan juices an additional 4 to 6 minutes. Pour pan juice over fish fillets and serve garnished with a cilantro sprig, a quarter of tomato, and a quarter of lemon.

Yield: 4 servings

Nutritional Analysis: Each serving provides 270 calories; 12 g fat; 31 g protein; 4 g net carbohydrate; 5 g dietary fiber; and 99 mg cholesterol.

Stuffed Lake Trout

Salmon or pike may be used in place of the trout in this recipe.
You will not need to scale the trout or salmon; however,
if using pike, it should be scaled. Remember never to overcook
fish as it will turn dry and chewy. The cherry tomatoes in the recipe
provide lycopene, one of the most potent carotenoid antioxidants.

---

1 cup (235 ml) 98 percent fat-free
  chicken broth

½ cup (98 g) quinoa or brown rice

2 tablespoons (28 g) omega-3-rich
  margarine

1 yellow onion, finely chopped

1 cup (100 g) mushrooms, sliced

2 teaspoons dried tarragon

Salt and pepper to taste

1 cup (175 g) cherry tomatoes, halved

2 tablespoons (28 ml) lemon juice

2 tablespoons (28 ml) canola oil

2 whole lake trout, cleaned

2 tablespoons (16 g) all-purpose flour

In a medium-size saucepan, bring chicken broth to a boil. Stir in quinoa or rice, cover, and reduce heat to low. Simmer 45 to 60 minutes, or until tender and all the broth is absorbed.

Preheat oven to 400°F (200°C, or gas mark 6), and line a baking sheet with parchment paper.

To prepare stuffing, melt margarine in a large skillet over medium heat. Sauté the onions and mushrooms until tender. Season with tarragon, and salt and pepper to taste. Add cherry tomatoes and sauté 1 to 2 minutes longer, stirring constantly. Remove from heat and mix with cooked quinoa or rice. Pour in lemon juice and toss.

Sprinkle the canola oil over the trout and inside the cavity. In a small bowl, mix together flour, salt, and pepper. Coat the inside and outside of the trout with the flour mixture. Fill trout with the stuffing mixture.

Bake uncovered for 10 minutes per inch of fish, or until the fish flakes easily with a fork.

Yield: 4 servings

Nutritional Analysis: *Each serving provides 440 calories; 19 g fat; 37 g protein; 25 g net carbohydrate; 3 g dietary fiber; and 94 mg cholesterol.*

Thai-Style Fish and Seafood Chowder

Coconut oil contains a significant amount of saturated fat, so it should be used only occasionally, and in smaller amounts. Whiting or codfish may be used to substitute for the tilapia in this recipe. Cilantro is easily grown in an herb garden, and is considered to be mildly anti-inflammatory, containing beta-carotene and vitamin K. Lemongrass is rich in folate and zinc.

---

3 cups (705 ml) 98 percent fat-free chicken broth

10 small baby red potatoes, diced

3 cobs fresh sweet corn, cooked, kernels removed

¾ cup (175 ml) coconut milk

½ teaspoon fresh ginger, minced

1 teaspoon dried lemongrass

1 teaspoon green curry paste (increase to 1 tablespoon [15 g] for spicier flavor)

½ cup (45 g) napa cabbage, finely chopped

Four 5-ounce (140 g) tilapia fillets

2 tablespoons (15 g) fish sauce

¾ cup (150 g) fresh shrimp, deveined, with tails on

¾ cup (150 g) bay scallops

¼ cup (15 g) fresh cilantro, chopped

In a large saucepan, heat chicken stock over high heat until it reaches a boil. Reduce heat and add potatoes, sweet corn, coconut milk, ginger, lemongrass, curry paste, and cabbage. Cover and simmer for 15 minutes, stirring occasionally.

Add fish fillets and fish sauce, and cook for 5 minutes. Add shrimp and cook for another 2 to 3 minutes. Add scallops and cook 4 to 5 minutes longer, or until scallops are opaque. Sprinkle with fresh cilantro.

Yield: 6 servings

Nutritional Analysis: Each serving provides 485 calories; 10 g fat; 41 g protein; 54 g net carbohydrate; 7 g dietary fiber; and 115 mg cholesterol.

Wilted Spinach Salad with Teriyaki Salmon

This wonderful blend of flavors from the Mediterranean goes well with warm rolls or a slice of fresh bread. Spinach contains a flavonoid called kaempferol, which is associated with reduced risk of developing ovarian cancer.

4 salmon fillets
(4 to 5 ounces [115 to 140 g] each)
1 cup teriyaki (235 ml) marinade
1 large sweet onion
Canola oil spray
1 tablespoon (14 g) molasses
or brown sugar

¼ teaspoon salt
One 15½-ounce (435 g) can white beans
½ cup (70 g) pine nuts
½ cup (80 g) raisins
4 cups (80 g) fresh spinach
4 tablespoons (60 ml) reduced-calorie oil
and vinegar dressing

Marinate the salmon fillets for 20 to 30 minutes in the marinade.

To caramelize the onion, peel and slice onion into very thin slices. Spray a skillet liberally with canola oil and cook the onion slices over low heat 15 to 20 minutes, stirring occasionally. Onions should be soft and caramel-colored. Stir in molasses and salt. Remove from heat.

Heat the white beans in a small pan until boiling. Lower heat and simmer 1 to 2 minutes, remove from heat, and drain. In a dry pan, lightly toast the pine nuts until golden brown. Add raisins and brown for 1 more minute, stirring occasionally. Set aside.

Grill salmon 6 to 8 minutes per side over medium heat. (If you prefer, salmon can be broiled. Heat the broiler and place the fillets on a broiler pan, skin-side down. Broil 3 inches [7.5 cm] from the heat for 8 to 12 minutes.) Salmon should be opaque and flaky but not dry. Spray a large skillet with canola spray and add the spinach. Cook the spinach just until it wilts, stirring constantly. The spinach should appear very dark green in color. Remove from heat and immediately transfer onto serving plates.

Divide the spinach between 4 serving dishes. Sprinkle each with white beans and raisin-pine-nut mixture. Decorate with caramelized onions and crown with a salmon fillet. Drizzle each serving with a tablespoon of dressing.

Yield: 4 servings

Nutritional Analysis: Each serving provides 590 calories; 26 g fat; 37 g protein; 48 g net carbohydrate; 8 g dietary fiber; and 65 mg cholesterol.

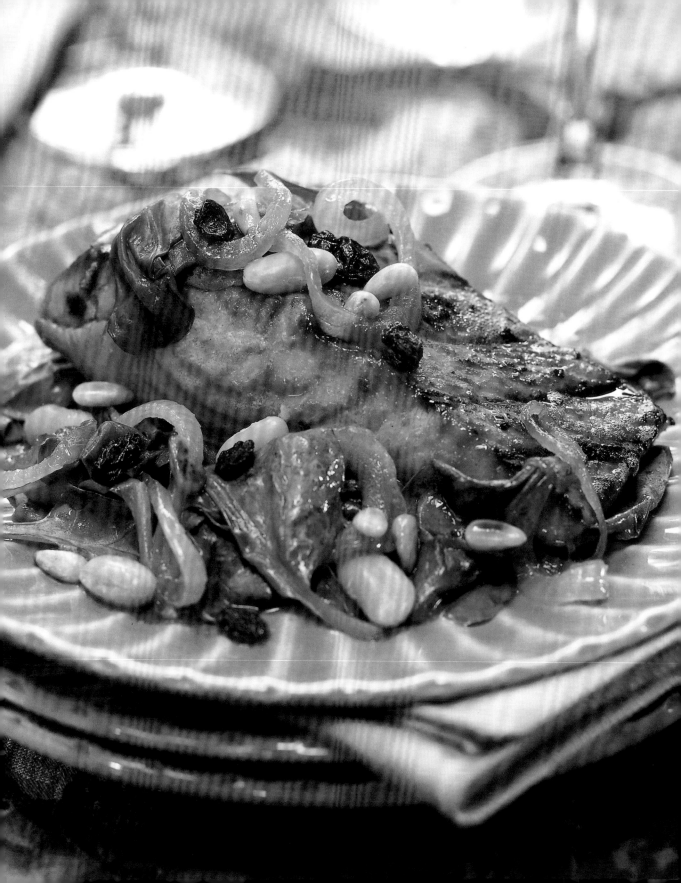

Tuna Salad Sushi

Choose canned light tuna over albacore, for reduced mercury content.
Seaweed contains known anti-inflammatory nutrients,
including eicosapentaenoic acid (EPA), folate, and vitamin K.

¾ cup (175 ml) water

½ cup (100 g) sushi rice

1 teaspoon rice vinegar

1 teaspoon sugar

½ teaspoon salt

One 7-ounce (195 g)) can tuna,
  packed in water, drained

1 tablespoon (14 g) light mayonnaise

1 cucumber, peeled

2 nori seaweed sheets
  (about 7¼ × 8 in [18 × 20 cm])

Low-sodium soy sauce and wasabi paste,
  optional

Using a cooking pot with a tightly fitting lid, bring water to a boil over high heat. Add rice, cover, and reduce heat. Simmer 18 to 20 minutes, turn off heat, and allow the rice to stand for 10 minutes. Place rice in a large mixing bowl, and sprinkle with vinegar, sugar, and salt. Mix with a wooden spoon, and allow rice to cool.

In a small bowl, mix together the tuna and mayonnaise. Slice the cucumber in thin slices lengthwise. Cut each slice into long strips.

Prepare each sushi roll as follows: Place 1 seaweed sheet on a clean, dry surface or bamboo mat, shiny side down, with the longer side across the top and bottom. Place 1/2 cup (83 g) cooked rice onto the seaweed, and carefully spread evenly over the sheet, leaving 1 inch (2.5 cm) exposed at the right edge. Place strips of cucumber in a straight line in the middle of the rice, parallel to the exposed edge. Spoon half of the tuna onto the rice, forming a line next to the cucumber.

Carefully roll so as not to tear the seaweed, starting at the left edge, ending just before the right edge. Tuck rice in at the edges of the roll. Run a wet finger along the exposed edge of the seaweed, and complete rolling, pressing down to seal the edge to the roll. Slice into pieces 3/4-inch (2-cm) wide, using a sharp, slightly wet knife.

Serve with low-sodium soy sauce and wasabi (Japanese horseradish) if desired.

Yield: About 20 pieces of sushi (4 servings of 5 pieces each)

Nutritional Analysis: Each serving provides 200 calories; 5 g fat; 15 g protein; 21 g net carbohydrate; 1 g dietary fiber; and 17 mg cholesterol.

CHAPTER 2

Add-In Antioxidants

These days we hear a lot about antioxidants and how important they are for good health. But what are they, really? Antioxidants are chemicals that prevent or interrupt certain types of chemical reactions in the body. Thousands, even millions, of chemical reactions are happening in your body all the time. Some of these reactions involve the transfer of electrons from one molecule to another, creating unstable molecules, called free radicals, that are damaging to the body. Free radicals can damage or destroy cells, proteins, and even our basic genetic material, DNA. Diseases linked to free-radical damage include cancer, heart disease, diabetes, arthritis, cataracts, and kidney disease. Exposure to pollution, radiation, tobacco smoke, and the sun generates higher levels of free radicals in the body. Even though our bodies have natural processes to deal with free radicals, these factors, along with aging, put stress on our capacity to handle free radicals.

Antioxidants have the ability to stabilize free radicals, preventing the damage they cause. Some examples of antioxidants are vitamin A, found in fortified dairy foods; vitamin C, naturally occurring in citrus fruits; vitamin E, found in sunflower seeds, nuts, and oils; beta-carotene, found in orange foods such as carrots, sweet potatoes, cantaloupe, apricots, squash, and mangoes; lycopene, found in tomatoes, watermelon, guava, and pink grapefruit; and selenium, found in wheat, rice and Brazil nuts.

Phytochemicals

Phytochemicals are a group of compounds that can function as antioxidants. They are produced and stored in plants. There are many types of phytochemicals, and many ways in which they are beneficial to our health.

Cruciferous vegetables, such as cabbage, broccoli, broccoli sprouts, kale, and cauliflower, contain a phytochemical called sulforaphane. This phytochemical is thought to cleanse harmful compounds from the body, while boosting the body's own antioxidant defenses. Researchers have found that eating cruciferous vegetables is associated with a reduced risk of developing cancer, particularly lung cancer. Choose red cabbage over white because it has six to eight times greater antioxidant capacity.

FLAVONOIDS

Tea, chocolate, red wine, and many fruits and vegetables contain flavonoids, a type of phytochemical that can inhibit and even destroy many bacterial strains and viral enzymes in plants. Flavonoids are responsible for the distinctive color in many foods, such as the red in tomatoes and cherries, the purple in red cabbage and red onions, the yellow in squash and mangoes, and the blue in blueberries. These compounds have been shown to reduce the risk of cardiovascular disease and cancer, thus the recommendation to eat "five a day," meaning five or more servings of fruits and vegetables daily. Flavonoids are beneficial in other ways as well. For example, flavonoids found in lemons are anti-inflammatory, while those in apples have antidiabetic effects. It has long been known that cranberry juice is beneficial for urinary tract infections. Now we know that this is partly due to their flavonoid content.

ISOFLAVONES

Soy products are a rich source of a type of phytochemicals called isoflavones, which are thought to have a number of health benefits. Consumption of soy products may help to reduce blood pressure and LDL cholesterol (the bad cholesterol) in the blood. Soy may also improve the flexibility of the blood vessels, when twenty-five grams per day are consumed with a diet low in saturated fat and cholesterol. Moreover, soybeans are an excellent source of protein, fiber, calcium, and iron. They are also one of the few plant sources of omega-3 fatty acids.

PRESERVING PHYTOCHEMICALS DURING COOKING

To preserve the greatest phytochemical content in any cooked fruit or vegetable, you should avoid overcooking. Vegetables are best when cooked just enough to retain their bright color. Steaming or lightly sautéing are the best methods to use. In many fruits and vegetables, the skin contains the highest concentration of phytochemicals, so leave the skins on for optimal nutrient value and a greater fiber content. Fresh vegetables provide the best flavor; however, frozen vegetables are a good substitute. To get the greatest benefit, choose organically grown vegetables because their phytonutrient levels are higher than vegetables grown with conventional methods. Avoid canned vegetables as they tend to be high in salt and lower in the valuable phytochemicals and vitamins that fresh and frozen vegetables provide.

While it is true that eating more fruits and vegetables may cause you to spend a little more at the grocery store, clearly the health benefits are worth the cost. By adding more antioxidants to your daily diet, you will be making an investment in your future!

FYI
Research shows that individuals who drink two or more cups of tea per day have lower rates of heart disease and stroke. Preliminary studies show that the antioxidants in tea may also help to prevent skin cancer.

Butternut Squash Citrus Soup

Granny Smith apples are good to use in this recipe because of their firmness and tart flavor; however, you can substitute any green cooking apple. Apples are a good source of both soluble and insoluble fiber. One medium-size unpeeled apple provides over 3 grams of fiber, which is about 10 percent of the recommended daily fiber intake for adults.

---

2 tablespoons (28 ml) olive oil1 large
 yellow onion, thinly sliced
3 pounds (1.5 kg) butternut squash,
 peeled and cubed
2 Granny Smith apples, peeled, cored,
 and thinly sliced
¼ teaspoon ground coriander

¼ teaspoon ginger, finely chopped
2 cups (470 ml) vegetable broth
¼ cup (60 ml) orange juice
One 11-ounce (325 ml) can
 mandarin oranges, drained
Ground nutmeg for garnish

In a 6-quart (5.5 L) cooking pot, heat olive oil over medium heat, add onion, and sauté until the onion is slightly browned. Add squash and sauté for about 15 minutes. Add apple, coriander, and ginger, and sauté for an additional 2 to 3 minutes. Add vegetable broth and bring to a boil. Reduce heat to a simmer, and slowly stir in orange juice and mandarin oranges. Simmer 30 to 40 minutes, until squash is tender. Place soup in a blender or food processor, a little at a time, and purée until smooth. Reheat soup over low heat, if necessary. Add salt to taste and serve with a pinch of ground nutmeg sprinkled on top.

Yield: 6 to 8 servings

Nutritional Analysis: Each serving provides 165 calories; 4 g fat; 2 g protein; 29 g net carbohydrate; 5 g dietary fiber; and 0 mg cholesterol.

FYI
Selenium is classified as a "trace" mineral because the body needs less than 100 milligrams per day. Selenium helps protect cells from oxidative damage and might help relieve symptoms associated with rheumatoid arthritis. Plant foods contain selenium, as do nuts, certain meats, and seafoods. Supplements are not recommended unless blood tests show lower-than-normal levels of selenium.

Beet Salad with Port Wine Vinaigrette

If you plan to use canned mandarin oranges, make sure to remove them from the can before placing them in the refrigerator to chill because the can might impart an unpleasant metallic taste to the oranges. Beets contain a pigment that gives them their rich, purple-crimson color and is a powerful antioxidant. Beets are also a good source of folate and fiber, both of which are thought to help protect against heart disease.

---

3 small beets

2 tart green apples, diced

¼ cup (60 ml) port wine vinegar

⅓ cup (80 ml) extra virgin olive oil

2 tablespoons (8 g) orange zest

½ teaspoon salt

3 cups (60 g) mixed greens

¼ cup (30 g) walnuts, finely chopped

6 ounces (170 g) canned
     mandarin oranges, chilled

Boil beets until tender (25 to 30 minutes). Drain and place in the refrigerator to cool. Once the beets have reached room temperature, peel and dice them. In a large bowl, mix beets and apples.

Combine port wine vinegar, olive oil, orange zest, and salt in a blender and blend until smooth. Add to beet and apple mixture, gently tossing to coat well. Place in the refrigerator to chill for 2 to 3 hours.

Just before serving, place mixed greens on individual salad plates. Top with the beet-apple salad, sprinkle walnuts on top, and serve garnished with chilled mandarin oranges.

Yield: 6 servings

Nutritional Analysis: Each serving provides 215 calories; 16 g fat; 3 g protein; 13 g net carbohydrate; 4 g dietary fiber; and 0 mg cholesterol.

Napoleon Salad

Eggplant is a rich source of phenolic compounds, which are potent antioxidants.

For the vinaigrette:

¼ cup (115 g) extra virgin olive oil

⅛ cup (30 ml) balsamic vinegar

1 teaspoon crushed garlic

1 teaspoon ground mustard

Salt and pepper to taste

For the salad:

Canola oil spray

1 egg

2 cups (230 g) seasoned bread crumbs

⅛ cup (15 g) flaxseed, ground

1 teaspoon salt

1 medium-size eggplant, cut into ⅓-inch (8-mm) rounds

1 large tomato, sliced

⅔ cup (135 g) pine nuts, toasted

1 large yellow onion, cut crosswise into ¼-inch (6-mm) slices

2 ounces (55 g) goat cheese

4 cups (80 g) mixed greens

To make the vinaigrette : Combine all ingredients in a jar with a tightly fitting lid. Shake vigorously. Chill in the refrigerator 30 to 40 minutes.

To make the salad: Preheat oven to 325°F (170°C, or gas mark 3). Lightly spray a cookie sheet with canola oil.

Whisk egg until well blended, and pour into a pie pan or plate with raised edges. Mix bread crumbs, flaxseed, and salt, and place in a similar dish. Dredge each slice of eggplant in egg, and then in the crumb mixture. Bake eggplant in the preheated oven for 15 minutes, turn the slices over, and continue to cook for an additional 15 to 20 minutes, or until both sides are brown and crisp. Cover with aluminum foil, turn off the oven, and leave eggplant in warm oven while preparing salad.

Lightly spray a stovetop pan with canola oil and sauté onion slices until they are soft and lightly browned. Divide mixed greens evenly onto 4 salad plates.

For each salad, place an eggplant slice on top of the greens, and follow with a slice of tomato. Evenly sprinkle 1 ounce (28 g) of goat cheese on the tomato, and top with another slice of eggplant. Sprinkle pine nuts over each salad, and drizzle with balsamic vinaigrette.

Yield: 4 servings

Nutritional Analysis: Each serving provides 630 calories; 40 g fat; 17 g protein; 45 g net carbohydrate; 11 g dietary fiber; and 73 mg cholesterol.

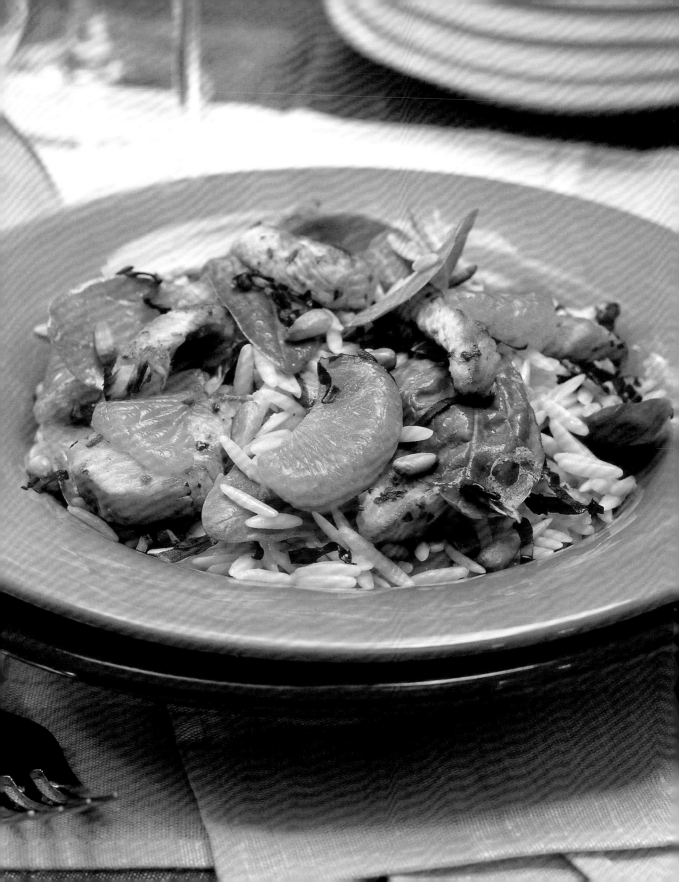

Fresh Spinach, Chicken, and Orzo Salad

Radicchio is Italian red-leafed chicory and is very low in calories—one cup (20 g) of shredded radicchio has just nine calories!

For the dressing:

2 tablespoons (28 ml) canola oil

2 tablespoons (28 ml) walnut or almond oil

1 tablespoon (14 ml) lemon juice

2 tablespoons (28 ml) orange juice

1 teaspoon lemon zest

1 teaspoon orange zest

1 teaspoon Dijon mustard

Salt and pepper to taste

For the salad:

1 quart (4 cups [950 ml]) water

1 cup (150 g) orzo

¼ teaspoon salt

1 tablespoon (14 ml) canola oil

Four 4-ounce (115 g) boneless, skinless chicken breasts, cut into 1-inch (2.5-cm) pieces

2 teaspoons minced garlic

1 tablespoon (4 g) oregano

½ cup (70 g) pine nuts, toasted

4 cups (120 g) fresh spinach, washed and stemmed

½ small radicchio, cored and finely shredded

One 11-ounce (325 ml) can mandarin oranges, drained

Combine all dressing ingredients in a jar with a tight fitting lid. Shake well. Chill in the refrigerator 30 to 40 minutes.

Bring the water to a boil in a large pot. Add orzo and salt, and return to a rapid boil. Cook 8 to 10 minutes. Drain and set aside.

Heat canola oil in a large skillet over medium-high heat. In a bowl, sprinkle garlic and oregano over chicken. Brown chicken in oil 2 to 3 minutes, then reduce heat to low. Cover and sauté 8 to 10 minutes, or until cooked through. Remove from heat and set aside.

Toss together spinach, radicchio, pine nuts, orzo, and chicken. Serve in individual dishes, garnished with mandarin oranges. Drizzle citrus dressing over top.

Yield: 4 servings

Nutritional Analysis: Each serving provides 630 calories; 32 g fat; 35 g protein; 50 g net carbohydrate; 4 g dietary fiber; and 63 mg cholesterol.

Butternut Squash Casserole

Butternut squash is pear shaped and sweet tasting. The bright, orange-colored flesh is due to the beta-carotene content, the same pro-vitamin that is found in carrots. Beta-carotene has been shown to have powerful antioxidant and anti-inflammatory properties.

For the squash:

2 pounds (1 kg) butternut squash

Canola spray oil

2 egg whites

1½ tablespoons (20 ml) nonfat milk

1½ teaspoons canola oil

½ cup (12 g) sugar substitute

2 tablespoons (28 g) omega-3-rich
  margarine, melted

1 teaspoon vanilla extract

⅓ cup (80 ml) soy milk

½ teaspoon ground cinnamon

⅛ teaspoon ground nutmeg

For the topping:

¼ cup (55 g) omega-3-rich margarine,
  melted

⅓ cup (75 g) light brown sugar

½ cup (12 g) sugar substitute

½ cup (60 g) all-purpose flour

½ cup (80 g) dried cranberries

1 cup (125 g) walnuts, chopped

Preheat oven to 375°F (190°C, or gas mark 5).

With a sharp knife, cut the squash in half and remove the seeds. Place cut side down in a baking pan sprayed with canola oil. Add 1/4 inch (6 mm) of water to the pan. Cover with foil and bake for 40 minutes, or until tender. Remove from oven and set aside until squash is cool enough to handle. Scoop out pulp with a spoon and mash. Reduce oven temperature to 350°F (180°C, or gas mark 5).

In a large mixing bowl, whip together the egg whites, nonfat milk, and canola oil. Blend in sugar substitute, margarine, vanilla, soy milk, and spices. Add mashed butternut squash and mix well. Spread evenly in a large casserole dish. Bake uncovered for 45 minutes. Remove from oven.

In a small bowl, combine topping ingredients. Sprinkle over casserole, and return casserole to oven for 8 to 10 minutes, until slightly browned on top.

Yield: 8 to 10 servings

Nutritional Analysis: Each serving provides 275 calories; 17 g fat; 6 g protein; 26 g net carbohydrate; 3 g dietary fiber; and 0 mg cholesterol.

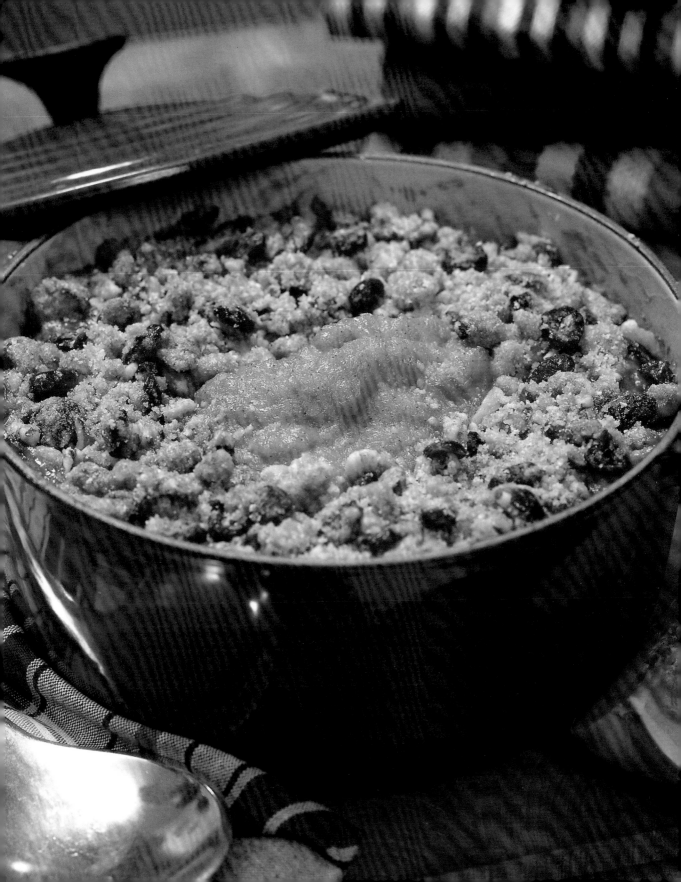

Potato Veggie Salad

Potatoes are a good source of vitamin C, providing about 25 percent of the adult recommended daily value per cup. They also contain a variety of phytonutrients that function as antioxidants in the body, including carotenoids and flavonoids. To boost this recipe even more, add a half cup (65 g) of finely chopped baby carrots.

For the dressing:

2 teaspoons cornstarch

2 teaspoons Dijon mustard

⅔ cup (160 ml) cold water

⅓ cup (80 ml) apple cider vinegar

1 teaspoon garlic, minced

½ teaspoon paprika

½ teaspoon Worcestershire sauce

For the salad:

2 pounds (1 kg) small red potatoes

2 ounces (55 g) broccoli sprouts

½ cup (60 g) celery, finely chopped

½ cup (65 g) red onion, finely chopped

To make the dressing: Mix together cornstarch, mustard, and water in a small sauce pan. Bring mixture to a boil and cook 2 to 3 minutes, until mixture thickens. Remove from heat and allow to cool completely. In a blender or food processor, combine cooled cornstarch mixture with remaining dressing ingredients, and blend until smooth. Put in refrigerator to chill.

To make the salad: Cook potatoes in boiling water until tender (about 20 minutes). Remove and set aside to cool. When cool enough to handle, dice and place in a large mixing bowl. Add in broccoli sprouts, celery, and red onion. Toss gently to combine. Gently stir in the dressing.

Yield: 8 servings

Nutritional Analysis: Each serving provides 95 calories; 0 g fat; 3 g protein; 18 g net carbohydrate; 2 g dietary fiber; and 0 mg cholesterol.

Chicken Vegetable Soup with Lemongrass

Fresh corn on the cob is sweeter and more tender than the canned or frozen varieties and can be used in any recipe that calls for corn. Buy the corn still in its husk, strip off the husk, and remove the silk. Using a sharp knife, cut along the cob lengthwise, removing several rows at a time. Corn is a good source of thiamin, fiber, folate, and vitamin C.

Two 14-ounce (390 g) cans 98 percent fat-free chicken broth

Four 4-ounce (115 g) boneless, skinless chicken breasts, cubed

1 red bell pepper, cored, seeded, and diced

1 yellow bell pepper, cored, seeded, and diced

3 ears fresh corn on the cob, kernels removed

3 to 4 stalks of celery, finely chopped

1½ teaspoon fresh lemongrass, finely chopped

½ teaspoon crushed red pepper

In a medium-size pot, bring the chicken broth to a boil. Reduce heat and add the chicken breast. Simmer for 30 minutes. Add remaining ingredients, and cook for an additional 10 minutes, until bell peppers are just tender. Serve with whole-grain bread or crackers.

Yield: 4 servings

Nutritional Analysis: Each serving provides 220 calories; 5 g fat; 32 g protein; 10 g net carbohydrate; 3 g dietary fiber; and 73 mg cholesterol.

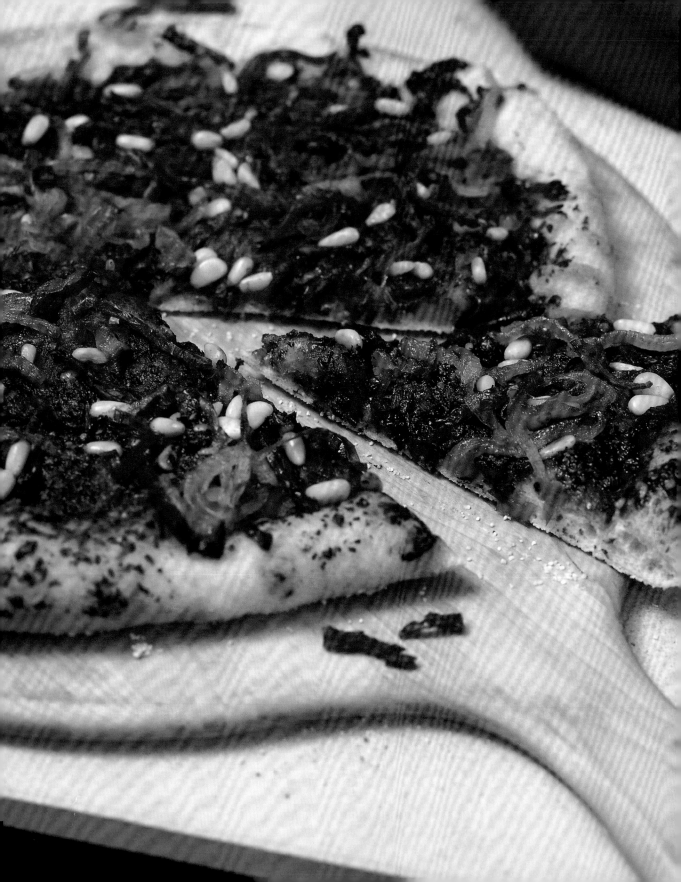

Caramelized Onion Pizza
with Basil and Pine Nuts

For a quicker version of this tasty pizza, toss all the dough ingredients into a breadmaking machine (set to the "dough only" setting). Pizza dough can be made in advance and refrigerated for 1 to 2 days, then brought to room temperature prior to use. For a sweeter pizza, replace sun-dried tomatoes with golden raisins that have been sautéed for 1 to 2 minutes with the onions.

For the dough:

2½ teaspoons active dry yeast (1 packet)

1 cup (235 ml) very warm water
   (about 105°F [40°C])

1¾ (210 g) cups all-purpose flour, divided

1½ cups (180 g) whole-wheat flour

¼ cup (30 g) ground flaxseed

1/2 teaspoon kosher salt

2 tablespoons (28 ml) extra virgin olive oil

2 teaspoons honey

Olive oil spray

For the topping:

1 cup (50 g) chopped sun-dried tomatoes,
   packed without oil

½ cup (20 g) fresh basil, chopped

¼ cup (60 ml) plus 2 tablespoons (28 ml)
   extra virgin olive oil, divided

¼ cup (25 g) grated Parmesan cheese

2 large Vidalia onions, thinly sliced

2 teaspoons sugar

Olive oil spray

½ cup (120 g) tomato paste

½ cup (70 g) pine nuts, toasted

To make the dough: In a small bowl, whisk together the yeast and warm water. Let stand until foamy (about 5 minutes). In a large bowl, combine 1½ cups (180 g) of the all-purpose flour, the wheat flour, flaxseed, and salt.

Whisk the olive oil and honey into the yeast mixture. Slowly add the yeast mixture to the flour mixture, stirring with a fork constantly, until the dough forms a slightly sticky ball. Lightly flour a smooth surface with the remaining flour. Knead the dough on the surface until smooth and elastic, about 10 minutes. Form into 2 tight, smooth balls.

Spray the inside of a large bowl with olive oil spray. Place the dough balls in the bowl, and turn each one once, so that the top sides are lightly coated with olive oil. Cover the dish with a clean, slightly dampened dish towel, and let rise in a warm place until doubled in size, about 30 to 40 minutes.

(continued on next page)

To make the topping: Place the sun-dried tomatoes in a small amount of water for 10 minutes, or until softened. Place basil, 1/4 cup (60 ml) olive oil, and the Parmesan cheese in a blender. Process until smooth. In a skillet, heat the remaining olive oil over medium-low heat, and sauté the onions until they are soft and light brown (about 15 minutes). Stir in sugar, and continue cooking for another 1or 2 minutes. Remove from the pan and set aside.

To make the pizza: For the best crust, preheat the oven to 450°F (230°C, or gas mark 8), and preheat a pizza stone for about 30 minutes. Divide the pizza dough into 2 portions. For each pizza, place a dough ball on a lightly floured surface, and sprinkle a little flour on top. Using your fingertips, flatten the dough ball to a thick round. Using a rolling pin, roll out the dough until it is about 1/4-inch (6-mm) thick, turning and lightly flouring as needed to keep the dough from sticking. Turn the edges of each round to form a slight rim.

Spray the surface lightly with olive oil spray. Carefully slide the dough onto the preheated pizza stone. Spread half of the tomato paste and half of the basil mixture over the top of the dough. Scatter half of the sun-dried tomatoes, onion, and pine nuts evenly over the top, leaving 1/2 inch (1 cm) around the edge free of topping.

Bake at 450°F (230°C, or gas mark 8) until the crust is golden brown, 8 to 10 minutes. Slice on a cutting board with a pizza knife and serve.

Yield: Two 14-inch (35-cm) pizzas (4 servings per pizza)

Nutritional Analysis: Each serving provides 450 calories; 24 g fat; 11 g protein; 46 g net carbohydrate; 7 g dietary fiber; and 2 mg cholesterol.

Cool Cranberry-Grape Salad

This recipe has been adapted from one my grandmother prepared every holiday. My sister, Eloise, has carried on the tradition with her own version, which I have adapted slightly here. Cranberries are high in flavonoids, which are pigments with a high antioxidative capacity, as well as vitamin C. Cranberries have long been associated with prevention of urinary tract infections and may be beneficial in preventing peptic ulcers.

One 12-ounce (340 g) bag cranberries

2 large bunches red seedless grapes, halved (about ⅔ of a pound [305 g])

One 12-ounce (340 g) can pineapple chunks, packed in unsweetened juice

8 ounces (225 g) walnuts, chopped

3 apples, cored, and diced

One 12-ounce (340 g) container nonfat whipped topping

½ cup (12 g) sugar substitute

8 ounces (225 g) mini-marshmallows

Place bag of cranberries in freezer for at least 2 hours. Put frozen cranberries in a blender or food processor and process until finely chopped. In a large bowl, mix cranberries with grape halves, pineapple chunks, walnuts, and apples. In a separate bowl, mix together the nonfat whipped topping and sugar substitute. Add to cranberry mixture, stirring gently. Add in mini-marshmallows. Chill for 30 minutes before serving.

Yield: 10 to 12 servings

Nutritional Analysis: Each serving provides 270 calories; 13 g fat; 6 g protein; 33 g net carbohydrate; 4 g dietary fiber; and 0 mg cholesterol.

FYI
Consuming antioxidant supplements can be detrimental, depending on their content. For example, vitamin A toxicity can occur with excessive amounts of the preformed vitamin, causing severe illness and even death. The best way to get your antioxidants is from food sources, not pills.

Fresh Mango and Melon Salsa

To get the most out of a mango, stand the mango on its end, stem side down, to determine the alignment of the pit. Cut along both sides of the pit (so you're cutting the biggest slice possible), from top to bottom, with a sharp knife. Take each mango half and score the flesh lengthwise and crosswise, making sure not to cut through the peel. Cut away the pieces from the peel. Take the center piece, removing any additional peel, and make slanted cuts along the pit to remove the remaining flesh.

---

2 mangoes, slightly firm, peeled and cubed

1 kiwi fruit, peeled and diced

½ cantaloupe, seeded and diced

½ red bell pepper, finely chopped

2 tablespoons (28 ml) lemon juice

1 teaspoon balsamic vinegar

2 teaspoons extra virgin olive oil

1 small jalapeno pepper, finely chopped

Salt and pepper to taste

In a medium-size mixing bowl, combine all ingredients. Place in refrigerator and chill for 2 hours. Serve with any grilled white fish or as an appetizer with crackers.

Yield: 8 to 10 servings

Nutritional Analysis: Each serving provides 55 calories; 1 g fat; 0 g protein; 10 g net carbohydrate; 2 g dietary fiber; and 0 mg cholesterol.

Herbed Carrots with Ginger Vinaigrette

Ginger has been popular in China for thousands of years, used both as a medicine and to flavor food. It is thought to have anti-inflammatory properties and has long been used for calming an upset stomach. When combined with carrots, high in beta-carotene, and oranges, the result is a great anti-inflammatory dish!

---

2 large oranges

1 teaspoon orange zest

2 tablespoons (28 ml) balsamic vinegar

2 tablespoons (28 ml) white wine vinegar

⅓ cup (80 ml) extra virgin olive oil

½ teaspoon salt

2 tablespoons (40 g) honey

½ teaspoon ginger, minced

One 16-ounce (455 g) package baby carrots

¼ cup (30 g) walnuts, chopped

Juice the oranges and place the juice in a blender or food processor. Add the orange zest, vinegars, olive oil, salt, honey, and ginger and process until smooth. Place baby carrots in a medium-size saucepan, cover with dressing, and stir to coat. Cover pan and cook on medium heat for 10 minutes, stirring occasionally. Remove from heat. Stir in walnuts and serve.

Yield: 6 to 8 servings

Nutritional Analysis: *Each serving provides 175 calories; 13 g fat; 2 g protein; 14 g net carbohydrate; 2 g dietary fiber; and 0 mg cholesterol.*

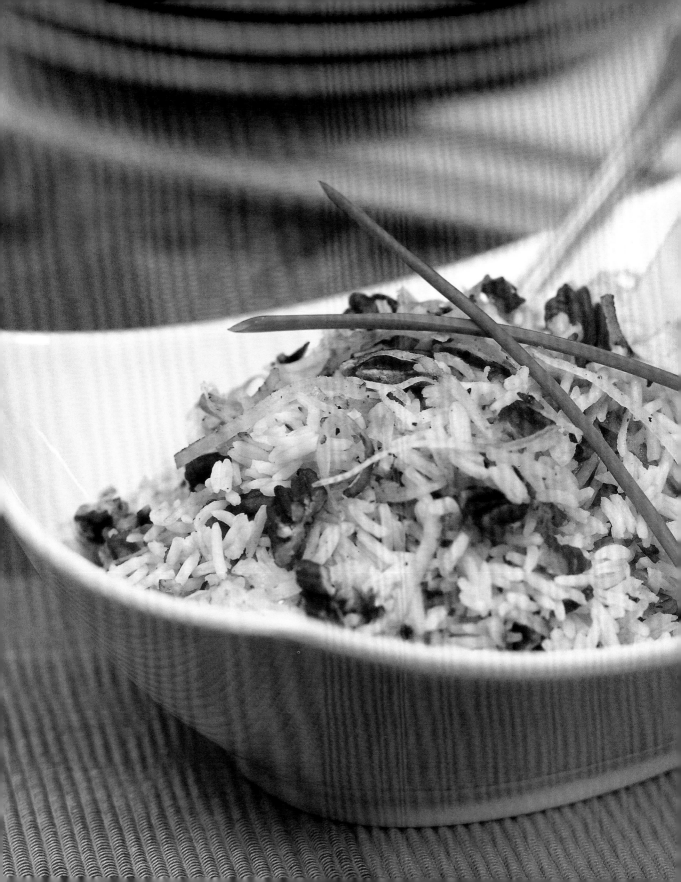

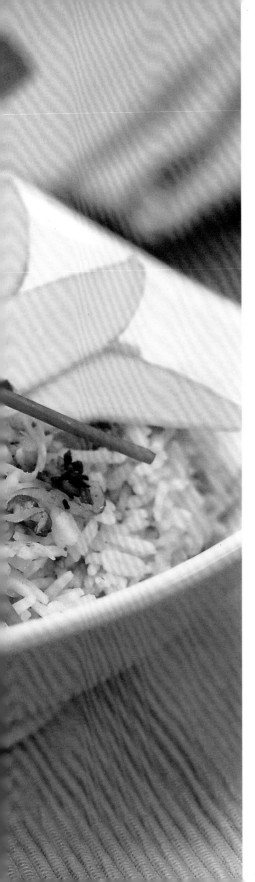

Mango Pecan Rice

Mangoes are packed with vitamin A, known to have antioxidant properties and important to the immune system. A great alternative to the long-grain rice in this recipe is brown rice. Though it takes a bit longer to cook than white rice, brown rice is rich in fiber and selenium, a trace mineral that is a component of antioxidant enzymes.

---

1 cup (185 g) long-grain rice

2 cups (470 ml) water

½ cup (60 g) pecan halves, chopped

½ cup (35 g) shredded sweetened coconut

⅓ cup (80 ml) mango juice

Salt to taste

1 mango, peeled and sliced lengthwise

Place rice and water in a medium-size cooking pot and bring to a boil. Turn down and simmer until liquid is completely absorbed, about 20 minutes.

In a large skillet, toast the pecan pieces until slightly browned. Add coconut and toast, stirring constantly, another minute until coconut is slightly browned. Add mango juice, cooked rice, and salt to taste. Mix well and serve topped with mango slices.

Yield: 4 servings

Nutritional Analysis: *Each serving provides 375 calories; 15 g fat; 5 g protein; 53 g net carbohydrate; 3 g dietary fiber; and 0 mg cholesterol.*

Mediterranean Stuffed Tomatoes

Hummus is one of the oldest foods that dates back to ancient Egypt.
It is made from chickpeas (also called garbanzo beans), which are rich
in protein, vitamins, minerals, and soluble fiber. These delicious tomatoes
make a great vegetarian main dish or side dish. Using home-cooked
chickpeas will result in a creamier taste, but canned chickpeas are a quicker
alternative. You can replace the olives with a variety of ingredients,
such as chopped roasted red pepper or spinach.

For the hummus:

One 16-ounce (455 g) can of chickpeas

¼ cup (60 ml) liquid from the canned
chickpeas

4 tablespoons (56 ml) lemon juice

1½ tablespoons (22 g) tahini

2 teaspoons garlic, finely minced

¾ cup (75 g) kalamata olives, pitted
and finely chopped

½ teaspoon salt

2 tablespoons (28 ml) olive oil

For the stuffed tomatoes:

8 whole, medium-size tomatoes

Two 4-ounce (115 g) sleeves
of soda crackers

8 sprigs fresh cilantro

8 lemon wedges

Combine chickpeas, reserved liquid, lemon juice, tahini, garlic, olives, salt, and olive oil in a food processor or blender. Process on a low setting for 3 to 5 minutes, stopping often to stir mixture, until the mixture is smooth and creamy. Set aside.

Cut a thin slice off the top of each tomato. Scoop out and discard the insides. Crush the soda crackers with a rolling pin or in a food processor. Place in a medium-size mixing bowl and add the hummus. Mix well. Stuff each tomato with the mixture, and garnish with a sprig of cilantro. Serve with a lemon wedge.

Yield: 8 servings

Nutritional Analysis: Each serving provides 260 calories; 11 g fat; 7 g protein; 30 g net carbohydrate; 6 g dietary fiber; and 0 mg cholesterol.

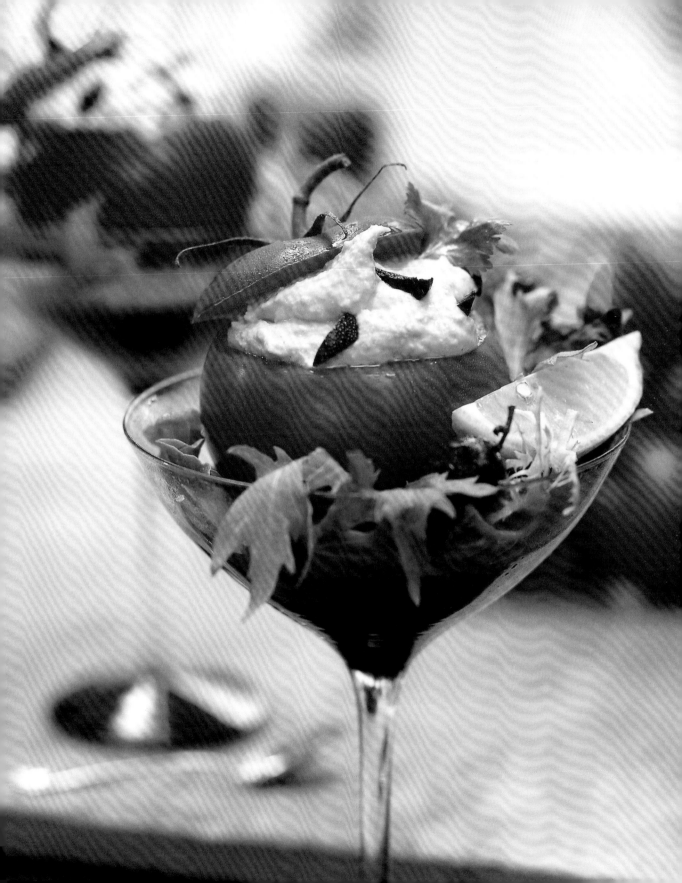

Pomegranate Green Bean Salad

Pomegranate seeds are a good source of antioxidants and entirely worth the effort of removing them from the fruit—just be sure to wear an apron because the juice may spurt out and stain your clothes. The best way to remove seeds is to cut off the crown and score the pomegranate husk lengthwise in four places. While holding the fruit under water in a large bowl, split the sections and separate the seeds from the husk. The seeds will sink to the bottom of the bowl, while the peel and membranes will float.

½ cup (50 g) pecan halves

2 pounds (1 kg) thin green beans, trimmed and halved

2 tablespoons (28 ml) extra virgin olive oil

2 tablespoons (28 ml) pomegranate juice

2 teaspoons (10 ml) apple cider vinegar

Salt and pepper to taste

¼ cup mandarin (60 ml) orange wedges, sliced into ½-inch (1-cm) pieces

¼ cup (55 g) pomegranate seeds

Preheat oven to 350°F (180°C, or gas mark 4). Spread pecan halves on a baking sheet, and toast in the oven until lightly browned (8 to 10 minutes), stirring often. Remove from oven, cool and chop coarsely.

Meanwhile, blanch green beans until they turn bright green and are barely tender, about 10 minutes. Rinse in cold water to stop the cooking process, and place in the refrigerator to cool further.

In a large mixing bowl, whisk together the olive oil, pomegranate juice, and vinegar. Season with salt and pepper to taste. Add cooled green beans, mandarin orange slices, and pomegranate seeds. Toss gently. Serve topped with pecan halves.

Yield: 8 servings

Nutritional Analysis: Each serving provides 125 calories; 9 g fat; 3 g protein; 6 g net carbohydrate; 5 g dietary fiber; and 0 mg cholesterol.

FYI

Pomegranate juice is a rich source of antioxidants, but consult your doctor if you plan to drink pomegranate juice daily because it can interfere with an enzyme in the liver that metabolizes medications. This may cause the level of certain medications in your blood to be higher than desirable and can lead to serious health problems. The same is true of grapefruit juice.

Parmesan Polenta Pie

Add fresh mushrooms to the sauté to provide additional fiber and B vitamins.

---

3 cups (705 ml) water, divided

1 cup (135 g) yellow cornmeal

½ teaspoon salt

¼ teaspoon black pepper, ground

¼ cup (25 g) grated Parmesan cheese

¼ cup (13 g) sun-dried tomatoes,
  chopped and soaked in water

1 egg white

2¼ teaspoons (12 ml) nonfat milk

2 teaspoons olive oil

Olive oil spray

2 tablespoons (28 ml) olive oil

1 medium-size yellow onion, finely diced

1 green bell pepper, diced

1 red bell pepper, diced

One 6-ounce (170 g) can tomato paste

2 tablespoons (8 g) fresh oregano
  (or ¼ teaspoon dried)

¼ teaspoon black pepper

2 medium-size tomatoes, sliced

One 6-ounce (170 g) can pitted black
  olives, sliced

To make the polenta, heat 2 cups (470 ml) of water over high heat in a medium-size cooking pot. In a mixing bowl, combine cornmeal, remaining 1 cup (235 ml) of cold water, and salt. Stir into the boiling water. Cook for 1 to 2 minutes, until the mixture thickens. Remove from heat and add black pepper, Parmesan cheese, and sun-dried tomatoes. Set aside to cool.

Beat egg white, nonfat milk, and olive oil together in a large mixing bowl. Add polenta by spoonfuls, blending well. Spray a 9-inch (22.5-cm) pie pan with olive oil. Spread the dough into the pie pan to form a thick crust. Let stand, uncovered, for 2 hours, until the crust dries.

Preheat oven to 350°F (180°C, or gas mark 4). Spray crust with olive oil and bake for 45 minutes.

Meanwhile, heat 2 tablespoons (28 ml) of olive oil in a skillet over medium-high heat. Sauté onion and bell peppers until onion turns translucent (3 to 4 minutes). Set aside.

Spread tomato paste over pie crust and sprinkle with oregano and pepper. Spread onion and bell peppers over the tomato paste, followed by the sliced tomatoes and olives. Place under broiler in the oven, using a middle rack. Broil 3 to 4 minutes. Serve hot.

Yield: 8 servings

Nutritional Analysis: Each serving provides 237 calories; 12 g fat; 6 g protein; 22 g net carbohydrate; 8 g dietary fiber; and 3 mg cholesterol.

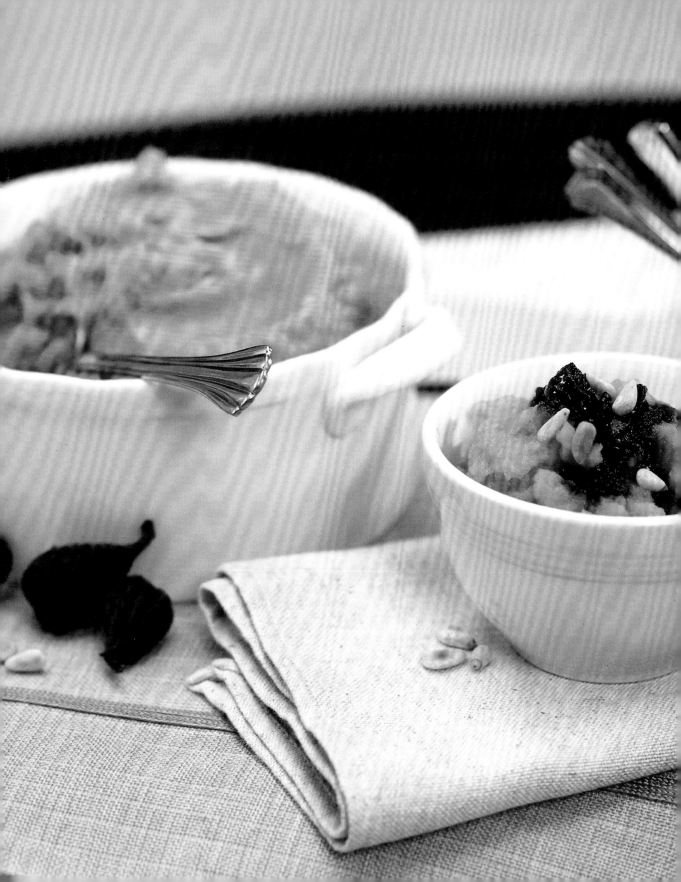

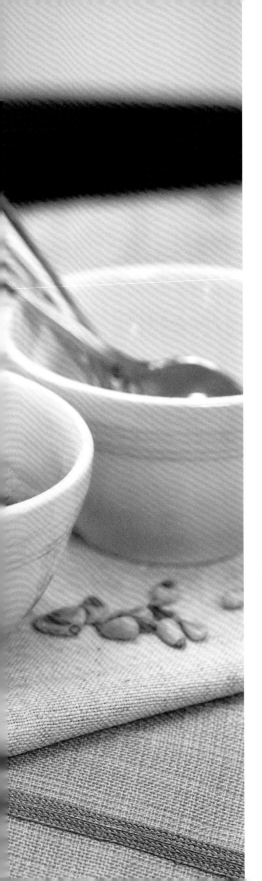

Parsnip Purée
with Balsamic Sauce

Parsnip has a sweet, nutty taste and is high
in soluble fiber, folate, and potassium.

¾ cup (175 ml) balsamic vinegar

8 soft dried figs, finely chopped

½ teaspoon garlic, finely chopped

½ cup (120 ml) water

½ teaspoon Dijon mustard

2 tablespoons (28 ml) extra virgin olive oil

½ teaspoon nutmeg

4 parsnips, peeled and cut into ¼-inch (6-mm) thick slices

2 medium-size sweet potatoes, peeled and cubed

3 tablespoons (40 ml) extra virgin olive oil

3 tablespoons (4.5 g) sugar substitute

Salt to taste

⅓ cup (45 g) pine nuts, toasted, optional

Boil vinegar in a small saucepan 3 to 4 minutes. Stir in the
next six ingredients, and heat on low 5 to 8 minutes, stirring
occasionally. Set sauce aside.

Boil parsnips and sweet potatoes until tender (15 to 18
minutes). Drain, reserving about ½ cup (120 ml) of water.
Place vegetables in a food processor or blender, along with
half of the reserved water, and process until smooth, adding
additional water as needed. Add olive oil, sugar substitute, and
salt to taste. Serve purée topped with fig sauce and pine nuts.

Yield: 10 servings

*Nutritional Analysis: Each serving provides 210 calories;
10 g fat; 2 g protein; 25 g net carbohydrate; 5 g dietary fiber;
and 0 mg cholesterol.*

Red Pepper and Olive Tapenade

This tapenade is delicious on rye or whole wheat crackers,
or added to hummus in a pita sandwich. If you are unable to get
pitted olives, first cut along one side of each olive, along the pit.
Turn and do this on all four sides, removing as much meat as possible.

---

2 red bell peppers, cored and cleaned

½ red onion

Olive oil spray

1½ cup (150 g) kalamata olives, pitted

3 tablespoons (26 g) capers, rinsed
    and drained

1 tablespoon (4 g) fresh parsley

¼ teaspoon lemon zest

1 teaspoon garlic

1 teaspoon black pepper, ground

Preheat broiler or grill. Cut off the tops of the bell peppers and halve lengthwise. Remove the seeds and membranes. Slice the red onion into large pieces. Place the pepper and onion pieces in a baking dish, spray olive oil generously over the pieces, and place on the upper rack of the oven. Roast under the broiler until the peppers blister and are tender. Set aside to cool. Once cool, slice the peppers and onion into strips.

Combine the red pepper, onion, and remaining ingredients in a food processor and process until mixture is finely chopped.

Yield: 12 to 16 servings of 2 tablespoons (30 g) each

Nutritional Analysis: Each serving provides 25 calories; 2 g fat; 0 g protein; 1 g net carbohydrate; 1 g dietary fiber; and 0 mg cholesterol.

Roasted Red Pepper Joes

I have offered two options for the sauce—use which ever you prefer.
Both are rich in lycopene, which comes from the tomato purée.

For sweet barbecue sauce:

2 tablespoons (28 ml) canola oil

1 onion, finely minced

1 teaspoon minced garlic

1 cup (250 g) tomato purée

1 cup (150 g) tomatoes, seeded and finely chopped

¼ cup (60 ml) cider vinegar

¼ cup (60 ml) apple juice

2 tablespoons (3 g) sugar substitute

2 tablespoons (28 g) brown sugar

1 tablespoon (9 g) chili powder, optional

Salt and pepper to taste

For savory barbecue sauce:

2 tablespoons (28 ml) canola oil

1 onion, finely minced

1 teaspoon minced garlic

1 cup (250 g) tomato purée

1 cup (150 g) tomatoes, seeded and finely chopped

½ cup (120 ml) red wine vinegar

1 tablespoon (14 ml) Worcestershire sauce

2 tablespoons (3 g) sugar substitute

2 tablespoons (9 g) chili powder, optional

Salt and pepper to taste

For the Joes:

Olive oil spray

1 pound (455 g) 93 percent fat-free ground beef

One 12-ounce (340 g) jar roasted red peppers, chopped

1 teaspoon thyme

1½ cups (375 g) barbecue sauce

4 whole-grain hamburger buns

To make the sauce: Heat the canola oil in a medium-size saucepan. Add onion, and cook until translucent. Add garlic and cook for 1 to 2 minutes. Add the remaining ingredients, and bring to a boil. Reduce the heat and simmer 12 to 15 minutes, stirring occasionally.

To make the Joes: Lightly spray a large skillet with olive oil. Brown ground beef over medium-high heat until completely cooked. Add roasted red peppers, thyme, and desired barbecue sauce. Serve over whole-grain buns.

Yield: 4 servings

Nutritional Analysis: Each serving provides 410 calories; 11 g fat; 30 g protein; 39 g net carbohydrate; 4 g dietary fiber; and 60 mg cholesterol.

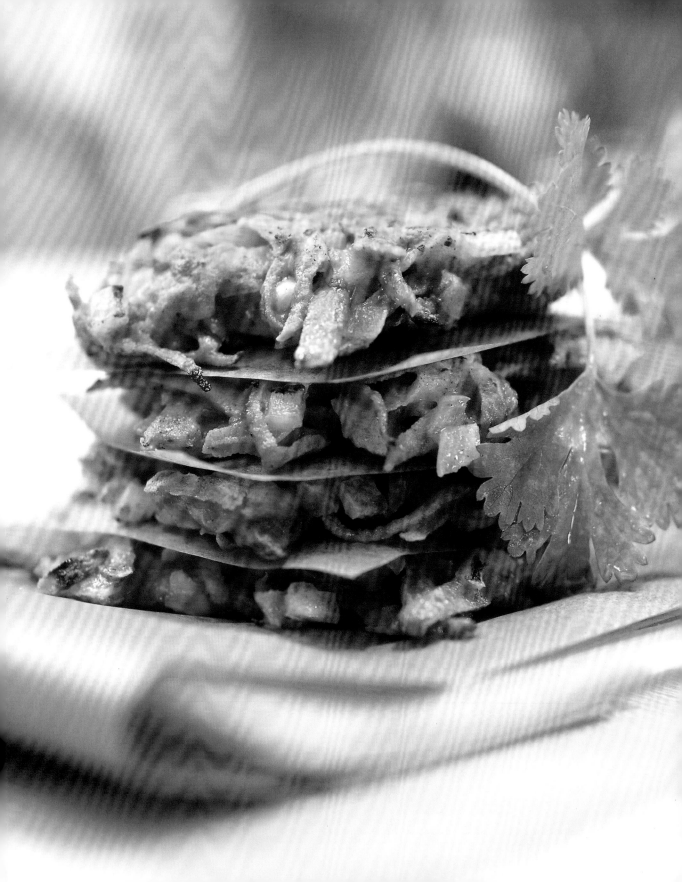

Savory Sweet Potato Latkes

Sweet potatoes are packed with beta-carotene and also contain vitamin C and manganese—all important antioxidant nutrients. There are more than 400 varieties of sweet potatoes, including the yam. They are best shredded with a grater or with a food processor.

---

2 sweet potatoes, peeled and coarsely shredded

½ yellow onion, finely chopped

⅓ cup (40 g) all-purpose flour

1 teaspoon kosher salt

1½ teaspoons curry powder

½ teaspoon cumin

½ teaspoon chili powder, optional

3 egg whites, beaten

¼ cup (60 ml) canola oil

¼ cup (15 g) fresh cilantro sprigs

Place shredded sweet potatoes between layers of paper towels and press down to squeeze out excess liquid. In a large bowl, mix together the shredded sweet potatoes, onion, flour, salt, and spices. Add egg whites and toss until mixture is well coated.

Heat canola oil in a large skillet over medium-high heat. Spoon sweet potato mixture into hot oil, using a large spoon. Flatten each latke with a spatula. Cook for several minutes on each side until golden. Drain on paper towels.

Garnish with cilantro sprigs.

Yield: 6 to 8 servings

Nutritional Analysis: Each serving provides 145 calories; 8 g fat; 3 g protein; 13 g net carbohydrate; 2 g dietary fiber; and 0 mg cholesterol.

Stir-Fried Marinated Tofu

Tofu is a great source of protein, making it an excellent choice to include in vegetarian diets. Four ounces (115 g) of tofu also provides about a third of the recommended daily value for iron, plus a substantial amount of omega-3 fatty acids and selenium, a nutrient important to the antioxidant system.

For the marinade:

¼ cup (60 ml) oyster sauce

¼ cup (60 ml) soy sauce

2 tablespoons (28 ml) water

1 teaspoon sesame oil

1 teaspoon ginger, minced

1 teaspoon garlic, minced

For the stir-fry:

1 pound (455 g) firm tofu

3½ tablespoons (50 ml) canola oil, divided

1½ tablespoons (12 g) sesame seeds

1½ cups (225 g) snow peas, trimmed

2 carrots, cut julienne-style

1 medium yellow onion, thinly sliced

15 ounces (420 g) baby corn

8 fresh shiitake mushrooms, sliced

Soy sauce to taste

Place all of the marinade ingredients in a bowl, and whisk together until well blended.

Drain tofu and cut into slices. Place in a shallow baking dish and coat with marinade. Cover and refrigerate for 3 hours or overnight, turning occasionally.

Preheat oven to 350°F (180°C, or gas mark 4). Meanwhile, heat 1 tablespoon (14 ml) of canola oil in a skillet to medium-high heat. Sauté tofu slices until browned on both sides. Return to baking dish and bake 8 to 10 minutes. Remove from oven and set aside, covered to keep warm.

Heat another 1½ teaspoons (7 ml) of canola oil in a skillet over high heat. Add sesame seeds and sauté until seeds turn golden (about 1 minute). Remove the seeds and place on a paper towel to drain. Heat the remaining oil. Add the snow peas, carrots, onion, baby corn, and mushrooms, and stir-fry 3 to 4 minutes, until snow peas turn bright green. Add soy sauce and sesame seeds. Toss well.

Place on a serving dish, and top with marinated tofu.

Yield: 3 to 4 servings

Nutritional Analysis: Each serving provides 360 calories; 18 g fat; 16 g protein; 30 g net carbohydrate; 6 g dietary fiber; and 0 mg cholesterol.

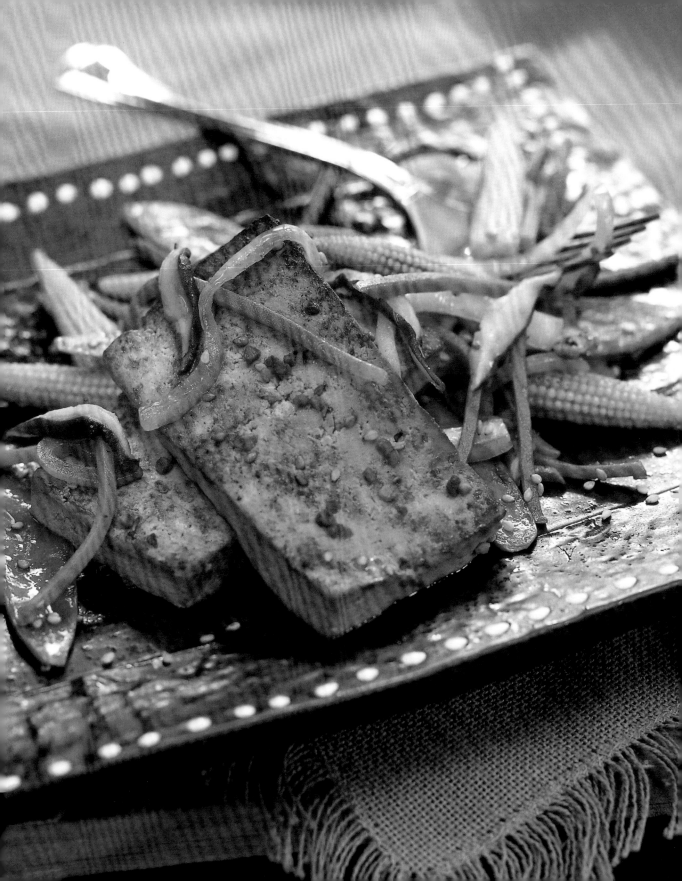

CHAPTER 3

Fabulous Fiber

A great deal has been written about fiber, and by now most of us know that fiber is good. Fiber consumption contributes to regularity and reduction of blood lipid levels, and it improves the body's regulation of blood sugar. Even so, the average American consumes just 15 grams or less of fiber per day, significantly below the current recommendation of 25 grams per day for women and 38 grams per day for men; or, for adults, 14 grams of fiber for every 1,000 calories consumed. For children between the ages of 1 and 3, aim for 19 grams of fiber; 25 grams for those 4 to 8 years of age.

Types of Fiber

INSOLUBLE FIBER

Most people know about insoluble fiber, or "roughage," as it is commonly called. This type of fiber does not dissolve in water and includes the nondigestible parts of plants such as bran, celery strings, fruit and vegetable skins, and so forth. Eating roughage is like taking your digestive tract to the gym for a good workout because it pushes against the intestinal wall while moving through, thereby strengthening the intestinal muscles.

SOLUBLE FIBER

Many people are less knowledgeable about soluble fiber. This type of fiber dissolves in water and forms a gel, slowing passage of food through the digestive system. Oatmeal, lentils, barley, dried beans, pectin fruits (such as apples), citrus fruits, and strawberries are all good sources of soluble fiber. Diets high in fiber are associated with lower levels of inflammatory markers, such as C-reactive protein. Eating the daily recommended amount of fiber has been shown to lower this blood protein, indicating a decrease in inflammation.

Benefits of a High Fiber Diet

One study of more than 40,000 people showed that a diet high in dietary fiber was linked to a 40 percent lower risk of coronary heart disease, when compared with a low-fiber diet. High-fiber diets have also been shown to improve blood-sugar levels and reduce the risk of developing diverticular disease, a condition in which the inner wall of the intestine can become infected and inflamed. Another study involving more than 10,000 physicians found that those who ate whole-grain cereal seven or more times per week were 28 percent less likely to develop heart failure than those who did not eat it at all. Those who ate the cereal two to six times per week were 22 percent less likely to develop the disease.

Increasing fiber in your diet should be done carefully to give your body time to adjust. By increasing your fiber intake gradually over a period of several weeks, you can avoid the uncomfortable gastrointestinal symptoms that can occur with more sudden increases in fiber.

You will also need to make sure you are getting plenty of fluid to go with the fiber you consume. Fiber absorbs water, so it is important to increase your fluid intake to avoid constipation when increasing your fiber intake. Women generally need a total of nine 8-ounce (235 ml) glasses of fluid per day, while men are more likely to need twelve glasses.

All beverages count, even if they contain caffeine, because they provide valuable fluid for your body, but avoid excessive amounts of fruit juice because it is high in calories and natural sugar. For example, 8 ounces (235 ml) of orange juice contains the equivalent of 5 teaspoons (20 g) of sugar; and 8 ounces (235 ml) of grape juice contains 8 teaspoons (30 g) of sugar, the same as a 12-ounce (355-ml) regular soda.

FYI
Fiber is a carbohydrate, but our bodies lack the necessary enzymes to digest it. Cows and other animals have those enzymes, which is how they can get fat just by eating grass and hay!

Shopping for Fiber

A good way to evaluate foods in the grocery store for fiber content is to look on the food label and divide "Total Carbohydrate" by "Dietary Fiber." You'll want to choose foods with a carbohydrate/fiber ratio of 7:1 or less for the most healthful fiber intake. For example, a food that has 18 grams of carbohydrate and only 2 grams of fiber has a carbohydrate/fiber ratio of 9:1. A food that has 21 grams of carbohydrate and 3 grams of fiber has a carbohydrate/fiber ratio of 7:1 and is therefore a better choice.

Soy Products

Soybeans and soy products are a great source of fiber. Soy is low in sodium and saturated fat; cholesterol-free; and high in calcium, iron, fiber, and vitamins.

Moreover, soy foods help reduce the risk of heart disease, cancer, and osteoporosis, and contribute to the relief of menopausal symptoms when consumed as recommended. Even though a daily intake of 40 to 60 grams of soy is recommended, most Americans eat very little soy. You can increase your soy intake by adding cooked soybeans to soup, chili, and baked bean recipes. Or, sprinkle chilled cooked soybeans over a green salad. Use soy milk instead of cow's milk when making pudding, and replace one-fourth of any recipe's total flour with soy flour. Soy products have become much more readily available, so keep an eye out for them in your local grocery store.

Flaxseed

Flaxseed (also known as linseed) is a dark or honey-colored seed, slightly larger than a sesame seed. Flaxseeds are rich both in omega-3 fatty acids and fiber. In fact, 2 tablespoons (15 g) of flaxseed meal contain the same amount of soluble fiber as one medium apple. Flaxseed contains a specific kind of fiber called lignans, which also serve as valuable phytochemicals and are thought to have anti-tumor effects in the body. Ground flaxseed can be added to many bread recipes, and can be consumed mixed in juice. These days, milled flaxseed can be bought in many grocery stores, but the best way to consume flaxseed is to grind it just before use, using a standard coffee grinder. Read the chapter on omega-3s for more information about flaxseed.

FYI
Soybeans and other soy products are a great source of protein, calcium, iron, omega-3s, and fiber. Roasted soybeans are available in many stores. Just ¼ cup (25 g) provides 15 grams of protein and 7.6 grams of fiber (about 30 percent of the recommended daily value).

Whole Grains

You can also increase your daily fiber intake by increasing the amount of whole grains in your diet. Branch out and try new whole-grain ingredients such as amaranth, buckwheat, bulgur, kamut, millet, quinoa, and whole-grain cornmeal. You might be surprised at how much more fiber you can consume in a day!

Brown Rice Stuffed Bell Peppers

One cup (165 g) of brown rice provides 14 percent of the
average adult daily value for fiber.

4 red bell peppers

2 tablespoons (28 ml) extra virgin olive oil

2 cups (200 g) mushrooms,
  finely chopped

3 scallions, finely sliced

1 to 2 stalks of celery, finely chopped

1 cup (190 g) brown rice

2 cups (470 ml) vegetable broth

Salt and pepper to taste

One 28-ounce (830 ml) can
  crushed tomatoes

1 tablespoon (4 g) dried oregano

2 teaspoons dried basil

¼ teaspoon ground cayenne pepper

¾ cup (75 g) pecans, toasted and
  finely chopped

⅛ cup (10 g) Parmesan cheese, finely
  shredded, optional

Preheat oven to 350°F (180°C, or gas mark 4).

Cut off the tops of the bell peppers, and remove seeds and membranes. Steam for 3 to 4 minutes, until they turn bright in color. Remove from the pot, and set aside.

Heat olive oil in a large saucepan over medium-high heat. Add mushrooms and sauté until tender. Add scallions, celery, and uncooked brown rice, and sauté another 3 to 4 minutes, stirring constantly. Add vegetable broth, salt, and pepper. Cover, bring to a boil, reduce heat, and simmer 40 to 45 minutes, until tender.

Meanwhile, place crushed tomatoes, oregano, basil, and cayenne pepper in a small saucepan. Heat over medium-high heat, stirring often, until mixture begins to boil. Reduce heat to low and cook for another 2 to 3 minutes, stirring to blend flavors together. Remove from heat and set aside.

In a large bowl, combine cooked brown rice and pecans. Stuff the mixture into the red bell peppers. Spread ½ cup (120 ml) of the tomato sauce in the bottom of a baking dish. Stand the bell peppers upright in the dish, and pour the remaining tomato sauce over the tops. Set the bell pepper tops leaning against each pepper on the inside of the dish. Bake 30 to 40 minutes.

Serve sprinkled with Parmesan cheese and topped with bell pepper tops.

Yield: 4 servings

Nutritional Analysis: Each serving provides 450 calories; 25 g fat; 10 g protein; 43 g net carbohydrate; 10 g dietary fiber; and 2 mg cholesterol.

Asian Asparagus Salad

When purchasing asparagus, pick thin, firm spears over ones that are thick, wrinkled, or droopy because the thinner spears are more tender and flavorful. To keep asparagus crisp, store it in the refrigerator wrapped in a damp paper towel and placed in a plastic bag. Don't use canned asparagus for this dish as it has already been cooked in the canning process. Asparagus is a good source of fiber, vitamins A and C, and folate. You'll want to use it as soon as possible to preserve the vitamin C and folate content.

---

1 tablespoon (8 g) sesame seeds

1½ pounds (680 g) asparagus, trimmed

1½ tablespoons (20 ml) sesame oil, divided

1 scallion, thinly sliced

1 tablespoon (14 ml) soy sauce

½ tablespoon (7 ml) rice vinegar

2 teaspoons sugar substitute

½ cup (60 g) cashew nuts, roasted and chopped

In a dry skillet, toast the sesame seeds over medium-high heat for about 2 minutes, until slightly golden brown.

Slice the asparagus diagonally into 2-inch (5-cm) pieces. In a skillet, heat 1 tablespoon (14 ml) of sesame oil over medium-high heat. Add the asparagus and scallion, and cook 2 to 3 minutes, stirring constantly, until they appear bright green in color. Remove from heat and set aside to cool.

Whisk together the soy sauce, remaining sesame oil, vinegar, and sugar substitute in a medium-size mixing bowl. Add the asparagus, sesame seeds, and cashew nuts, and toss until all of the asparagus is coated.

Yield: 4 servings

Nutritional Analysis: *Each serving provides 190 calories; 14 g fat; 7 g protein; 8 g net carbohydrate; 5 g dietary fiber; and 0 mg cholesterol.*

Brocco-Sprout Veggie Salad with Pitas

Broccoli sprouts are a highly concentrated source of sulforaphane,
a compound that helps mobilize the body's natural cancer-fighting abilities
and reduces the risk of developing cancer. Brocco-sprouts are available
in many grocery stores and are great on sandwiches too!

For the dressing:

⅓ cup (80 ml) lemon juice

½ cup (120 ml) olive oil

¼ teaspoon Worcestershire sauce

¼ cup (25 g) Parmesan cheese,
  freshly grated

Salt and pepper to taste

For the salad:

2 ounces (55 g) broccoli sprouts

1 English cucumber (or 2 regular),
  quartered and sliced

1 yellow bell pepper, coarsely chopped

1 red bell pepper, coarsely chopped

½ pound (225 g) cherry tomatoes, halved

4 whole-wheat pita breads

Olive oil spray

Combine dressing ingredients in a blender and blend until smooth. Chill in refrigerator for 30 minutes.

In a large bowl, mix together the salad ingredients. Add the dressing and toss well.

Cut each pita into 6 to 8 wedges. Spray a large skillet with olive oil and heat over medium-high heat. Place pita wedges in skillet and heat until browned on both sides. Serve with salad.

Yield: 6-8 servings

Nutritional Analysis: Each serving provides 225 calories; 16 g fat; 5 g protein; 16 g net carbohydrate; 3 g dietary fiber; and 2 mg cholesterol.

FYI
Cruciferous vegetables such as broccoli, cauliflower, brussels sprouts, kale, cabbage, and bok choy (Chinese cabbage) are packed with fiber and phytochemicals. Research shows that cruciferous vegetables are protective against cancer and may be related to reduced inflammation and risk of cardiovascular disease and diabetes.

Chicken and Bean Tortilla Soup

If your tastes run hot, use two cans of green chiles. Chiles contain
a substance that is associated with reducing inflammation called
"capsaicin," a chemical that is also used topically as a pain-relieving agent.
Green chiles are milder than red chiles and add pungency to this dish.

---

1 tablespoon (14 ml) extra virgin olive oil

1 red onion, finely chopped

1 tablespoon (10 g) garlic, finely minced

Four 4-ounce (115 g) boneless,
skinless chicken breasts, cut into
1-inch (2.5-cm) cubes

2 teaspoons chili powder

1 teaspoon cumin

One 28-ounce (830 ml) can crushed
tomatoes

Two 14½-ounce (440-ml) cans
98 percent fat-free chicken broth

1 bay leaf

2 to 3 corncobs, cooked, kernels removed

One 4-ounce (115 g) can green chiles,
chopped

One 15-ounce (420 g) can dark red kidney
or black beans

4 or 5 small corn tortillas

Canola oil spray

⅓ cup (20 g) fresh cilantro, chopped

3 scallions, finely sliced

Heat a large pot over medium-high heat and pour in olive oil. Add onion and garlic, and sauté
1 to 2 minutes, stirring constantly. Add chicken cubes and sauté until chicken is just cooked
through. Add chili powder and cumin, and sauté for another 2 minutes. Add crushed tomatoes,
chicken broth, bay leaf, corn kernels, chiles, and kidney beans. Bring to a boil and reduce heat.
Simmer 20 minutes.

Meanwhile, cut tortillas into ¼-inch (6-mm) strips. Spread on a baking sheet, lightly sprayed
with canola oil spray, and place on the middle rack of the oven, under the broiler. Toast tortilla
strips for a few minutes until tops are golden, stir, and toast for 1 to 2 minutes longer, taking care
not to burn them.

Serve soup in bowls topped with tortilla strips, fresh cilantro, and scallions.

Yield: 8 to 10 servings

Nutritional Analysis: Each serving provides 315 calories; 4 g fat; 28 g protein;
31 g net carbohydrate; 14 g dietary fiber; and 39 mg cholesterol.

Southern Spiced Peaches

Peaches are high in soluble fiber, which is important for lowering blood cholesterol, and vitamins A and C, both important antioxidants. Nectarines can also be used in this recipe because they are essentially the same fruit without the fuzz. Peaches and nectarines do not ripen after picking, although they do soften and are prone to bruising, so you'll want to handle them with care.

⅓ cup (80 ml) water

3 tablespoons (40 ml) white wine vinegar

1⅓ cup (33 g) sugar substitute

2 whole cloves

1 teaspoon ground cinnamon

½ teaspoon nutmeg

2 pounds (1 kg) firm ripe peaches, pitted and sliced

Place water, vinegar, sugar substitute, and spices in a large pot. Bring to a boil over medium-high heat. Reduce heat and add peaches. Simmer 10 to 15 minutes. Remove from heat and place in a heat-resistant container. Cover and chill for at least 2 hours.

Yield: 8 servings

Nutritional Analysis: *Each serving provides 45 calories; 0 g fat; 1 g protein; 9 g net carbohydrate; 2 g dietary fiber; and 0 mg cholesterol.*

FYI
In the late 1970s, a study conducted by the Food and Drug Administration and the National Cancer Institute indicated that heavy consumption of saccharin, an artificial sweetener, might increase the risk of developing bladder cancer. Heavy consumption was defined as six or more servings of the sweetener, or two or more 8-ounce (235-ml) servings of saccharin-sweetened beverages daily. No greater risks were found for those consuming less than this amount.

Bruschetta with Black Bean Salsa

Black beans are an excellent source of folate, and rank at the top of the
scale when compared with other beans for antioxidant activity.
They are also high in fiber. You can include these power-packed legumes
in a wide variety of dishes, including Hispanic, Caribbean, Mediterranean,
and Asian dishes. If you don't have time to cook the beans from scratch, use
beans from a 15-ounce (420 g) can that have been rinsed and drained.

For the salsa:

1 cup (100 g) sweet white corn, cooked

1 English cucumber, finely chopped

1 cup (30 g) fresh spinach leaves,
stemmed and finely chopped

¼ cup (30 g) red onion, finely chopped

2 cups (450 g) black beans, cooked

1 large jalapeno pepper, seeded and
finely chopped

2 tablespoons (8 g) fresh cilantro,
finely chopped

3 tablespoons (40 ml) lemon juice

3 tablespoons (40 ml) extra virgin olive oil

½ teaspoon ground cayenne pepper,
optional

Salt and pepper to taste

For the bruschetta:

1 French baguette

Olive oil spray

Mix together salsa ingredients in a medium-size mixing bowl. Cover and let stand 10 to 15
minutes while preparing bread.

Slice the baguette into ½-inch (1-cm) slices, and lay out on a baking sheet. Spray lightly with
olive oil. Toast under oven broiler until lightly browned. Turn and toast other side, spraying
lightly with olive oil as for the first side. Serve with topping in a separate bowl, or placed on top
of each piece of toast.

Yield: 30 to 35 slices (10 to 12 servings)

*Nutritional Analysis: Each serving provides 75 calories; 1 g fat; 3 g protein; 11 g net carbohydrate;
4 g dietary fiber; and 0 mg cholesterol.*

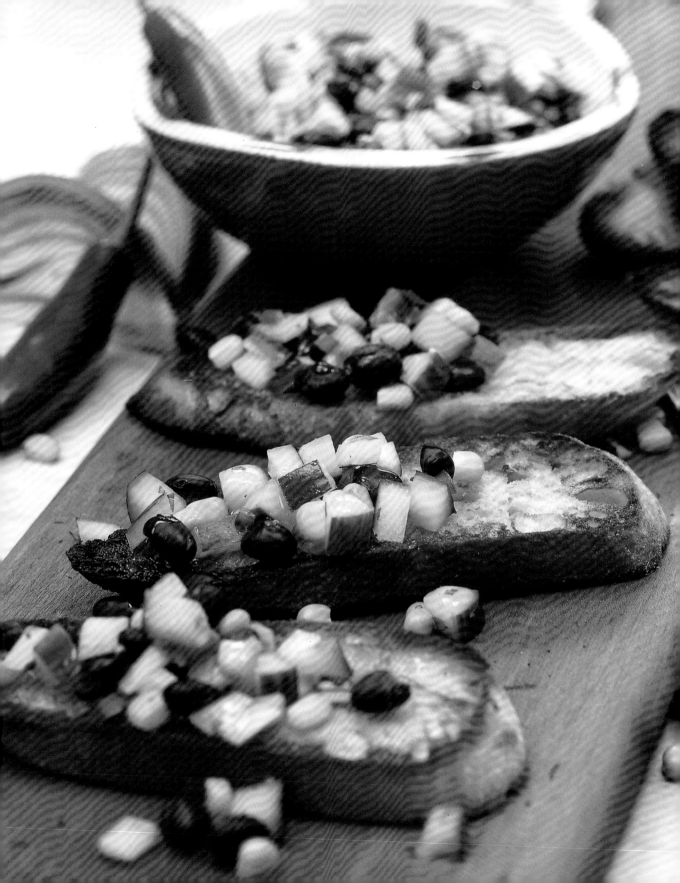

Creamy Mushroom
Spinach Soup with Quinoa

Quinoa is a food native to South America, once a staple of the Incas. Quinoa is high in protein and has an excellent amino acid profile. If you don't have quinoa in the pantry, barley is a good substitute to use in this dish.

⅔ cup (120 g) quinoa

3 tablespoons (40 g) omega-3-rich margarine

1 onion, finely diced

1 cup (100 g) fresh shiitake mushrooms, diced

8 ounces (225 g) cremini mushroom caps, diced

2 cups (60 g) fresh spinach

1 carrot, finely diced

3½ cups (820 ml) vegetable stock

1 cup (235 ml) fat-free half-and-half

Salt and pepper to taste

Fresh chives, chopped

In a dry skillet, toast the quinoa for 4 to 5 minutes over medium heat, stirring constantly. Set aside.

In a soup pot, melt margarine over medium-high heat and stir in onions. Sauté onions 5 to 6 minutes, stirring often. Add mushrooms and sauté another 2 to 3 minutes. Stir in quinoa, spinach, carrot, and vegetable stock. Bring to a boil, reduce heat, and simmer for about 20 minutes, until quinoa is tender.

Place soup in a blender and purée. Stir in fat-free half-and-half and return to soup pot. Reheat soup on low heat, without bringing to a boil. Season with salt and pepper, and serve garnished with chives.

Yield: 8 servings

Nutritional Analysis: Each serving provides 140 calories; 6 g fat; 4 g protein; 18 g net carbohydrate; 2 g dietary fiber; and 1 mg cholesterol.

FYI
Quinoa looks like a grain but is actually a seed. It comes from a South American plant with large leaves and a tall stalk with clusters of the seeds, which range in color from ivory to pink, red, brown, or black. You can use quinoa in many dishes as a substitute for grain, and it's high in protein, calcium, and iron.

Flaxseed Blueberry Walnut Pancakes

If you don't like blueberries, finely chopped fresh apples make a
great substitute in this delicious pancake recipe. For a healthful breakfast,
go easy on the syrup or use a sugar-free version.

1½ cups (180 g) all-purpose flour

½ cup (60 g) soy flour

2 teaspoons baking powder

1 teaspoon baking soda

½ teaspoon salt

⅓ cup (40 g) flaxseed, finely ground

½ cup (60 g) walnuts, finely chopped

2¼ cups (530 ml) reduced-fat buttermilk
or plain yogurt

½ teaspoon vanilla extract

2 eggs

1 cup (130 g) fresh or frozen blueberries,
thawed

Canola oil spray

Mix flours, baking powder, baking soda, and salt together with a fork, lifting upward to dissolve clumps and add air. Add in flaxseed powder and chopped walnuts. Whisk buttermilk, vanilla extract, and eggs together. Pour into flour mixture, add blueberries, and mix until just moistened. Mixture should be the consistency of thick batter. If needed, add a little water to achieve the right consistency.

Spray a large, nonstick skillet lightly with canola oil and heat over medium heat. For each pancake, pour ¼ cup (60 ml) of batter onto skillet. Cook until bubbles appear and edge of pancake appears dry. Turn and cook until golden brown. Serve warm.

Yield: 16 to 18 pancakes (5 to 6 servings)

Nutritional Analysis: Each serving provides 340 calories; 14 g fat; 15 g protein; 33 g net carbohydrate; 6 g dietary fiber; and 75 mg cholesterol.

(pictured on next page)

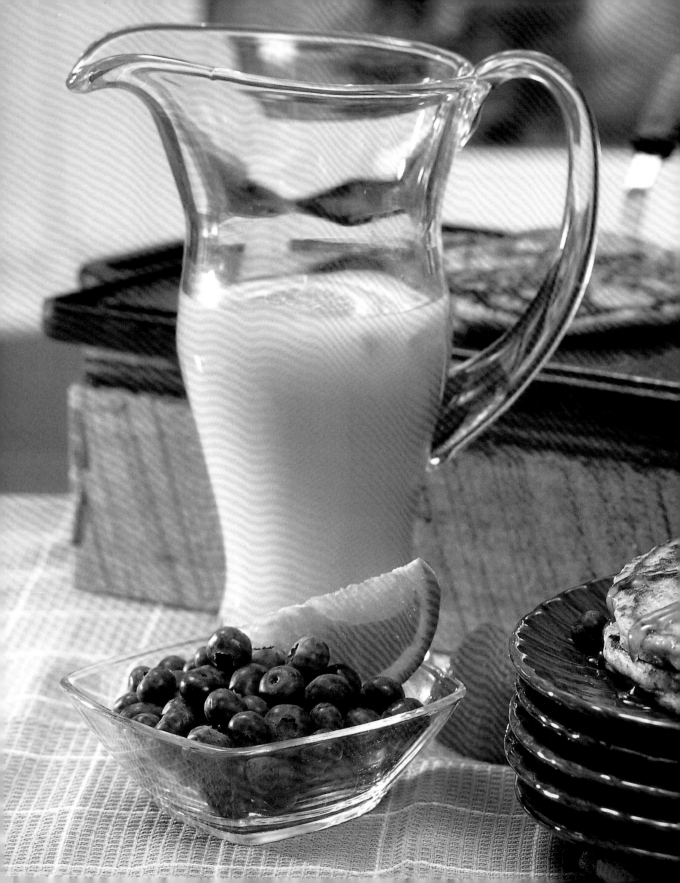

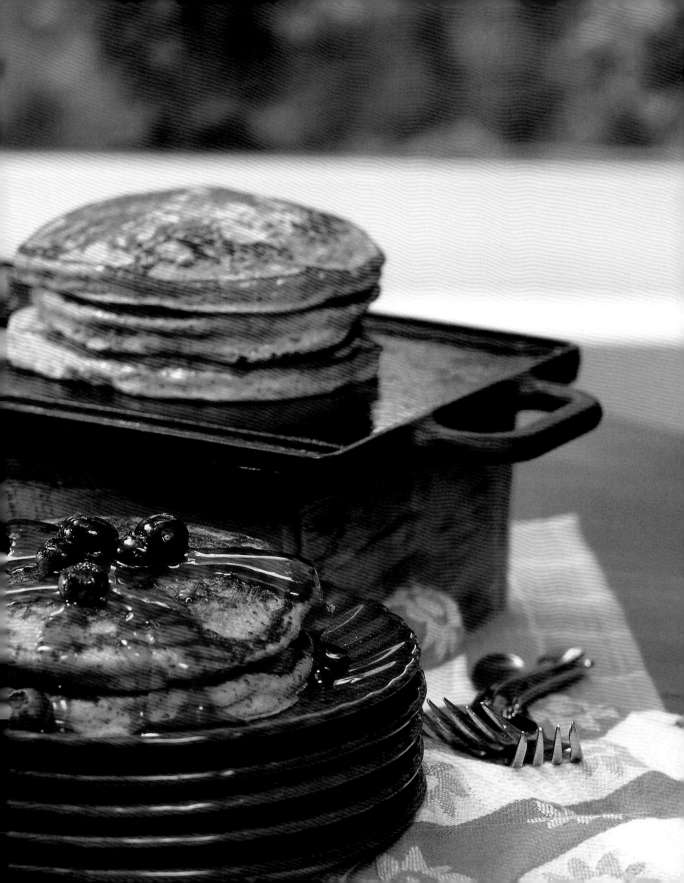

Healthy Hoppin' John

Hoppin' John is traditionally a Southern dish. I worked up this version as a healthful summer dish for my family. When choosing the avocado, pick one that is slightly soft to the touch, but not mushy. Avocados are rich in potassium and monounsaturated fat, as well as vitamin E and a type of carotenoids that protect against cancer.

One 15½-ounce (435 g) can black-eyed peas, drained

1 large tomato (or 4 plum tomatoes), diced

1 large mango, slightly firm, peeled and diced

1 yellow bell pepper, seeded, cored, and finely chopped

2 tablespoons fresh lime juice

1 avocado, slightly firm, peeled and diced

1 teaspoon garlic powder

¼ teaspoon ground cayenne pepper, optional

Salt to taste

In a large bowl, place black-eyed peas, tomato, mango, bell pepper, and lime juice. Mix until well blended. Add in diced avocado, garlic powder, and cayenne, and gently turn with a spoon to mix. Add salt to taste. Chill for at least 3 hours prior to serving.

Yield: 4 servings

Nutritional Analysis: Each serving provides 260 calories; 8 g fat; 11 g protein; 28 g net carbohydrate; 13 g dietary fiber; and 0 mg cholesterol.

FYI
If you eat five servings of fruits and vegetables, three servings of whole grain products, and three servings of any grain products per day, you will most likely achieve the 25 grams per day recommended for adults.

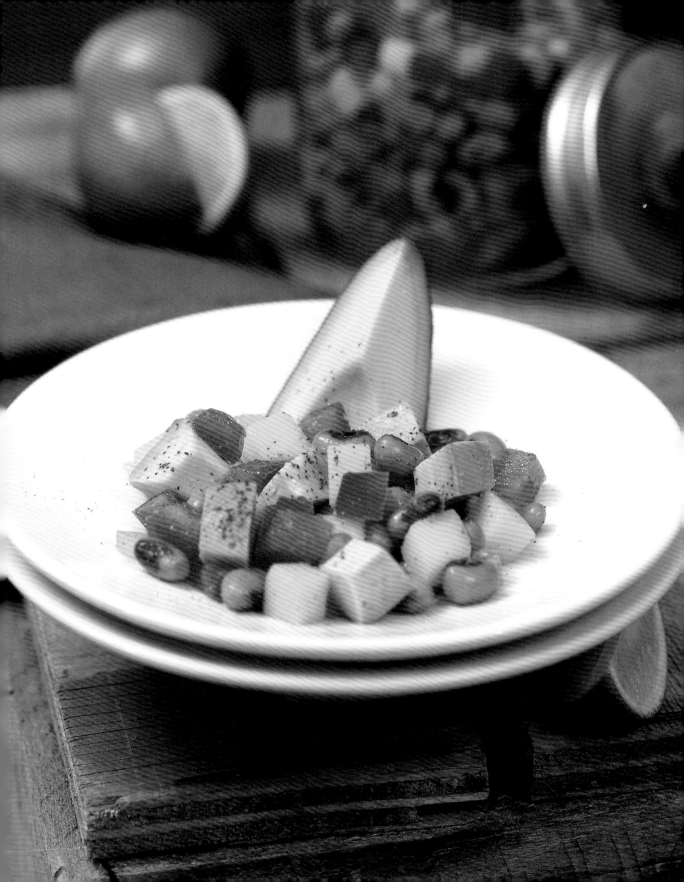

Mint Chutney Hummus

Although canned chickpeas do very well in this recipe, home-cooked
ones are smoother tasting and creamier. Using a slow cooker, cook the
dried beans in water, adding a clove of garlic for flavor, for eight
to ten hours on the low setting, until soft. Avoid adding salt before
they are fully cooked as the beans will not be as tender.

Two 14-ounce (390 g) cans of
chickpeas or 3½ cups (350 g)
home-cooked beans

3 tablespoons (40 ml) extra virgin
olive oil, divided

2 tablespoons (28 ml) lemon juice

1 teaspoon garlic, minced

⅔ cup (160 g) tahini

½ cup (50 g) fresh mint leaves, finely
chopped

1 green chile, seeded and finely chopped,
optional

½ teaspoon ground cumin

¼ teaspoon ground coriander

½ teaspoon salt

¼ teaspoon cayenne pepper

Drain half of the liquid from the chickpeas, and process in a blender or food processor to a
smooth purée. Add 2 tablespoons (28 ml) of olive oil and all remaining ingredients except
the cayenne pepper. Purée until smooth, stopping to mix ingredients with a spoon so that
the mixture is well blended. Transfer to a serving dish, create a swirl on top, and fill with the
remaining olive oil. Sprinkle cayenne pepper over the top and serve with whole-wheat pitas.

Yield: 8 servings

*Nutritional Analysis: Each serving provides 240 calories; 17 g fat; 8 g protein;
14 g net carbohydrate; 4 g dietary fiber; and 0 mg cholesterol.*

Curried Quinoa with Chickpeas and Okra

Okra is a great source of vitamin C. Just half a cup (50 g) provides about 20 percent of the average adult daily value. Okra also contains significant amounts of fiber, vitamin K, calcium, several minerals, and folate. It can be incorporated into most curry recipes, adding flavor and antioxidant capacity. For this recipe, frozen okra works well.

---

1 tablespoon (14 ml) canola oil

1 small onion, finely chopped

1 teaspoon cumin powder

1 teaspoon coriander powder

1 teaspoon curry powder

1 teaspoon garlic, finely minced

2 large carrots, finely diced

One 15-ounce (420 g) can chickpeas

1 cup (100 g) okra, stemmed and chopped

1 large tomato, diced

1 cup (184 g) quinoa

2 cups (470 ml) hot water

1 bay leaf

1 tablespoon (14 ml) lemon juice

Salt and pepper to taste

Heat oil in a medium saucepan over medium-high heat. Sauté onions until slightly browned, and reduce heat to medium. Add cumin, coriander, curry, and garlic, and sauté for 1 minute longer. Add carrots, chickpeas, okra, and tomato. Reduce heat and sauté for 5 to 8 minutes, stirring constantly.

Stir quinoa into vegetable mixture. Sauté 1 to 2 minutes. Add water, bay leaf, and lemon juice. Bring to a boil, cover, and reduce heat. Simmer for 15 to 20 minutes, until liquid is absorbed and quinoa is tender. Season with salt and pepper. Remove bay leaf before serving.

Yield: 6 servings

Nutritional Analysis: *Each serving provides 240 calories; 5 g fat; 8 g protein; 36 g net carbohydrate; 7 g dietary fiber; and 0 mg cholesterol.*

Onion and Jalapeno Corn Bread

Corn is a food that originated in the Americas, a staple of the native populations from ancient times. It is a good source of thiamin and folate, providing about 24 percent and 19 percent of the average adult daily values, respectively. Corn also provides fiber and several minerals. For the best results, use sweet, fresh corn on the cob, boiled briefly and cooled enough to allow you to cut the kernels from the cob.

½ cup (25 g) sun-dried tomatoes, chopped

1 medium-size onion, chopped

¼ cup (55 g) omega-3-rich margarine

1 cup (135 g) cornmeal

1 cup (125 g) all-purpose flour

3 tablespoons (4.5 g) sugar substitute

1 tablespoon (4.6 g) baking powder

½ teaspoon salt

2 egg whites

1 cup (235 ml) plus 1½ tablespoons (20 ml) nonfat milk, divided

1⅓ tablespoons (19 ml) canola oil

1 cup (100 g) corn kernels

1 jalapeno pepper, seeded and finely chopped, optional

1 cup (245 g) plain, nonfat yogurt

Canola oil spray

Preheat oven to 425°F (220°C, or gas mark 7). In a small bowl, combine sun-dried tomatoes and 1 cup (235 ml) of water, and soak for 15 minutes. Drain and set aside.

Sauté onion in margarine. Mix cornmeal, flour, sugar substitute, baking powder, and salt in a large mixing bowl. In a separate bowl, whip together egg whites, 1½ tablespoons (20 ml) nonfat milk, and canola oil. Add sautéed onion, margarine, and remaining milk. Mix well, and blend into the flour mixture. Add corn kernels, sun-dried tomatoes, jalapeno pepper, and yogurt, and mix until just combined. Pour into a casserole dish lightly sprayed with canola oil.

Bake 35 to 40 minutes, until a toothpick inserted into the center comes out clean. Cool for 10 minutes, remove from pan, and serve.

Yield: 10 to 12 servings

Nutritional Analysis: *Each serving provides 200 calories; 7 g fat; 6 g protein; 25 g net carbohydrate; 3 g dietary fiber; and 1 mg cholesterol.*

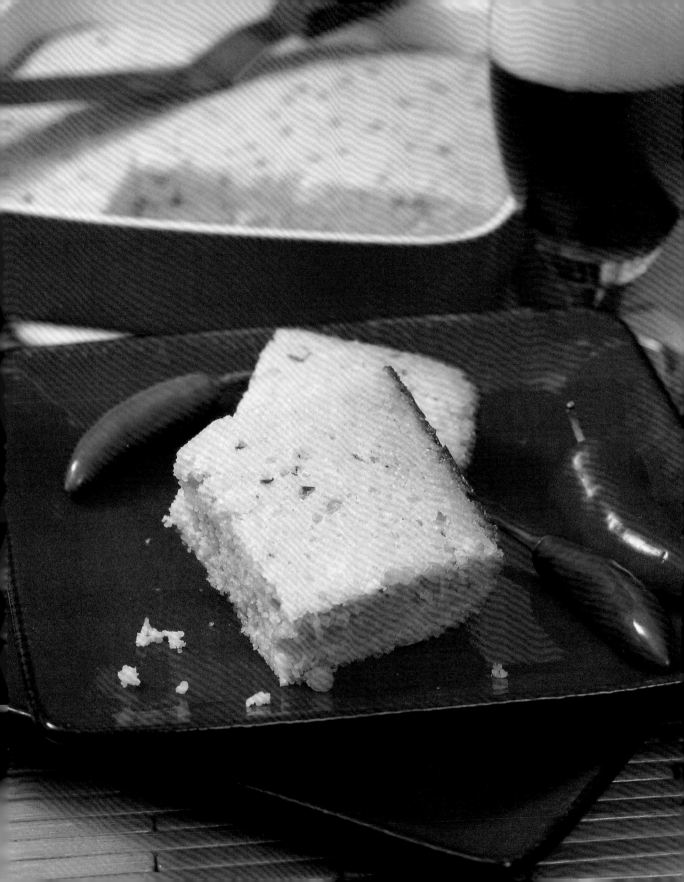

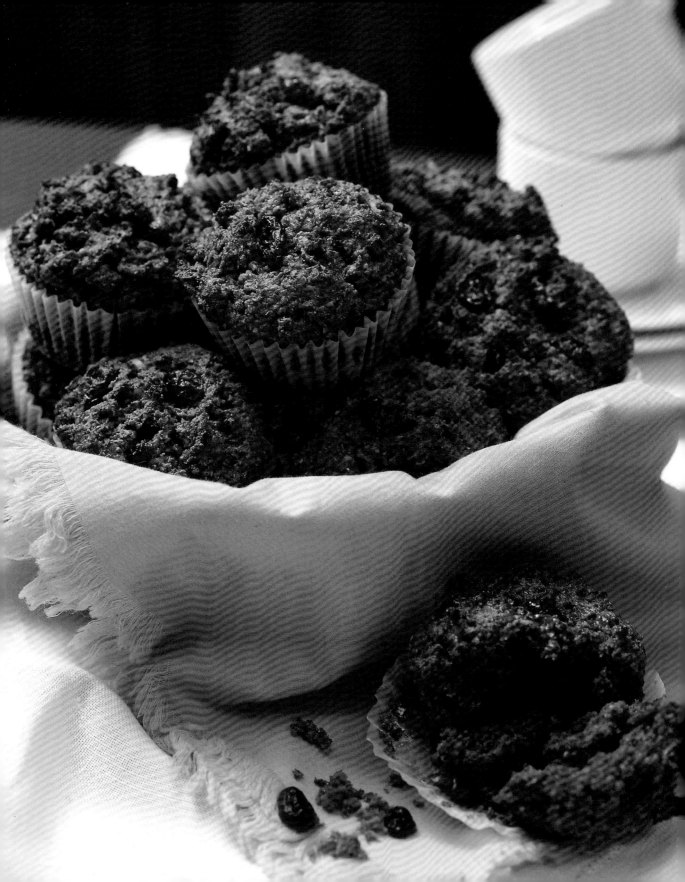

Orange-Cranberry Bran Muffins

These muffins are definitely for citrus lovers. The flaxseed
adds valuable fiber and antioxidants, as do the pecans and the bran.
For the best results, measure all of the ingredients carefully and
make sure the oven is preheated before you put in the muffins.
This will ensure that the muffins rise properly.

½ cup (60 g) soy flour

½ cup (60 g) whole-wheat flour

1½ teaspoons baking soda

Pinch of salt

¼ cup (30 g) flaxseed, finely ground

½ cup (50 g) bran

½ cup (80 g) sweetened dried cranberries

½ cup (60 g) pecans, finely chopped

⅓ cup (75 g) dark brown sugar

⅓ cup (8 g) sugar substitute

1 egg

¼ cup (60 ml) orange juice

2 tablespoons (8 g) grated orange zest

½ cup (120 ml) nonfat milk

⅓ cup (75 g) omega-3-rich
    margarine, melted

1 teaspoon orange extract, optional

Preheat oven to 400°F (200°C, or gas mark 6) and line a muffin pan with muffin cups. In a large mixing bowl, sift together soy flour, whole-wheat flour, baking soda, and salt. Stir in the flaxseed, bran, cranberries, pecans, brown sugar, and sugar substitute. Whip egg, orange juice, orange peel, and milk together in a separate bowl, and stir in melted margarine. Add orange extract, if desired. Add liquid blend to dry ingredients and stir until just moistened. Do not overmix. Spoon the batter into the muffin cups, filling them 3/4 full. Bake 15 to 20 minutes or until golden brown.

Yield: 16 muffins

Nutritional Analysis: Each muffin provides 125 calories; 8 g fat; 3 g protein; 11 g net carbohydrate; 2 g dietary fiber; and 12 mg cholesterol.

Quinoa Tabbouleh Salad

Quinoa, an ancient food from South America, is a high-protein staple and is referred to as "the Mother Grain of the Incas." It cooks like rice and can be prepared in a rice cooker with one part quinoa to two parts water.

---

2 cups (470 ml) water

1 cup (184 g) quinoa

¼ cup (60 ml) extra virgin olive oil

½ teaspoon sea salt

2 tablespoons (28 ml) lime juice

3 large tomatoes, diced

1 English cucumber, finely diced

3 to 4 scallions, thinly sliced

2 carrots, grated

1 cup (60 g) fresh parsley, finely chopped

¼ cup (25 g) fresh mint leaves, finely chopped

Bring water to boil in a medium-size sauce pan. Reduce heat and add quinoa. Cover and simmer 15 to 20 minutes, until quinoa is tender. Set aside to cool.

In a large bowl, combine remaining ingredients. Stir in cooled quinoa. Chill 1 to 2 hours before serving.

Yield: 6 to 8 servings

Nutritional Analysis: Each serving provides 175 calories; 9 g fat; 5 g protein; 19 g net carbohydrate; 4 g dietary fiber; and 0 mg cholesterol.

Ratatouille

Ratatouille is a popular Mediterranean vegetable dish with many variations. The dish is very flexible, so feel free to experiment by adding in other vegetables. You may want to try *herbes de Provence* for the seasoning as it will produce a more pungent flavor. If you have leftovers, ratatouille is great as a cold appetizer served on toasted slices of baguette.

---

1 eggplant, cubed

3 tablespoons (40 ml) extra virgin olive oil

1 red onion, thinly sliced

1 tablespoon (10 g) garlic, minced

4 large tomatoes, diced

1 red bell pepper, cored, seeded, and
   thinly sliced

1 yellow bell pepper, cored, seeded,
   and thinly sliced

3 zucchinis, sliced

½ teaspoon thyme

½ teaspoon oregano

1 teaspoon basil

1 tablespoon (4 g) parsley

Salt and pepper to taste

Lay eggplant cubes on paper towels and sprinkle with salt. Set aside for 30 minutes to allow them to drain off their bitter juices.

In a large saucepan, heat the olive oil over medium heat. Add onion and garlic, and sauté 2 to 3 minutes, stirring often. Add eggplant and sauté for another 2 to 3 minutes, stirring constantly. Add remaining ingredients, cover and cook 30 to 40 minutes, stirring regularly, until the vegetables are soft.

Yield: 4 servings

Nutritional Analysis: Each serving provides 185 calories; 11 g fat; 4 g protein; 13 g net carbohydrate; 9 g dietary fiber; and 0 mg cholesterol.

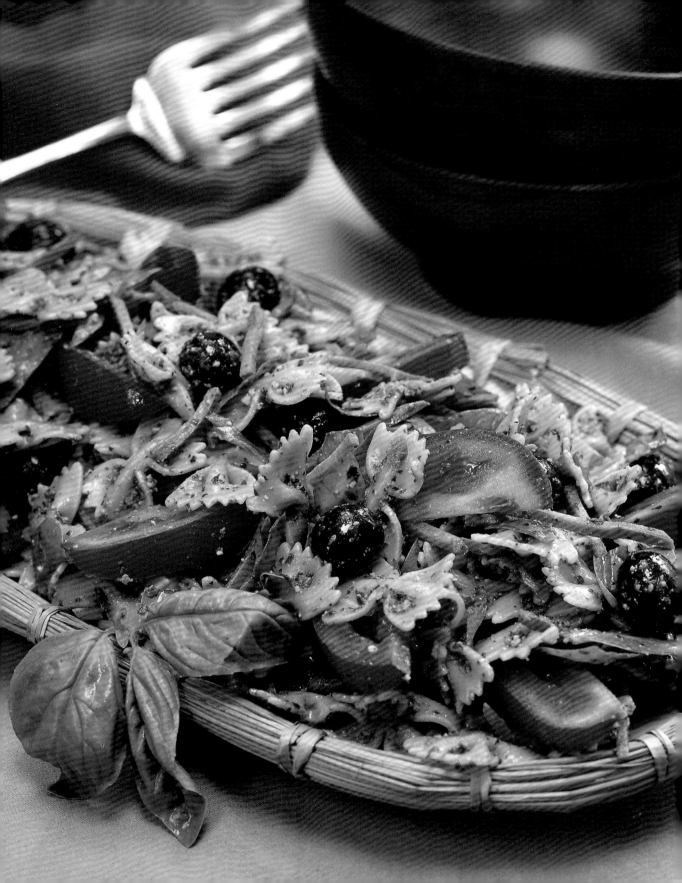

Springtime Pesto Pasta

Use whole-wheat pasta to boost this recipe's fiber content even higher. When cooking pasta, it's best to add it to the boiling water a little at a time, while stirring. Once the pasta is cooked, drain and rinse it with cold water to stop the cooking process and prevent the pasta from sticking together.

---

16 ounces (455 g) pasta
   (rotini, farfalle, or elbow)

Canola oil spray

1½ cups (60 g) fresh basil leaves

2 cloves fresh garlic

⅛ cup (30 ml) red wine vinegar

⅓ cup (80 ml) canola oil

½ cup (60 g) walnuts

1½ teaspoons salt

¾ cup (75 g) fresh Parmesan cheese, grated

One 4-ounce (115-g) can pitted black olives

4 plum tomatoes, chopped

¼ cup (30 g) fresh carrots, shredded

¼ cup (30 g) fresh red bell pepper, chopped

2 cups (60 g) fresh spinach, chopped

Bring 5 quarts (4.7 L) of water to a boil, and add pasta. Spray lightly with canola oil spray to keep pasta from sticking. Cook pasta until it is *al dente* (firm), rinse with cold water, and set aside to cool. Put basil leaves, garlic, red wine vinegar, canola oil, walnuts, and salt into a blender and blend on a low setting until consistency is smooth. You may need to stop the blender and stir the contents occasionally until the mixture blends well on its own. Place pasta in a large bowl and add pesto mixture and remaining ingredients. Mix well. Serve warm or chill 1 to 2 hours and serve as a salad.

Yield: 6 servings

Nutritional Analysis: Each serving provides 385 calories; 25 g fat; 14 g protein; 25 g net carbohydrate; 4 g dietary fiber; and 10 mg cholesterol.

Walnut Raisin Wheat Bread

This recipe can easily be made in your breadmaker. Add ingredients in the order listed, and choose the wheat bread setting. Because this bread does not contain any preservatives, you will need to store it in your refrigerator. (The wheat gluten in this recipe can be found in the baking section of most grocery stores.)

---

2 cups (470 ml) warm water, divided

4 teaspoons active dry yeast
  (1⅓ packets)

3½ cups (420 g) whole-wheat flour

2 cups (240 g) soy flour

2 teaspoons salt

2 tablespoons (12 g) wheat gluten

2 tablespoons (40 g) honey

3 tablespoons (40 ml) canola oil

½ cup (60 g) flaxseeds, finely ground

½ cup (60 g) wheat germ

½ cup (60 g) walnuts, chopped

½ cup (80 g) raisins

Canola oil spray

Dissolve yeast in 1 cup (235 ml) of water, slightly warm to the touch, and set aside for 5 minutes. Sift flours together with salt, and mix in the gluten powder. Mix the honey and oil with the remaining 1 cup (235 ml) of water, and add to the yeast mixture. Pour liquid into the center of the flour mixture, and blend well with a wooden spoon. In a small bowl, combine ground flaxseed, wheat germ, walnuts, and raisins. Add to flour mixture.

Place dough on a lightly floured surface and knead until dough is elastic. Shape into a smooth ball. Spray a glass bowl lightly with canola oil and place the dough in the bowl, lightly spraying the top of the dough with canola oil. Cover with a clean, damp paper towel. Leave to rise in a warm place until dough is doubled in size, about 1 hour.

Punch down the dough, form into a loaf, and place in a 5 × 9-inch (13 × 22.5-cm) loaf pan lightly sprayed with canola oil. Let rise a second time until doubled in size, about 45 minutes.

Preheat oven to 400°F (200°C, or gas mark 6). Bake until loaf is slightly brown on top, about 35 to 40 minutes. Remove from pan and let cool on a rack.

Yield: 1 loaf (about 14 servings)

Nutritional Analysis: Each serving provides 250 calories; 10 g fat; 11 g protein; 28 g net carbohydrate; 8 g dietary fiber; and 0 mg cholesterol.

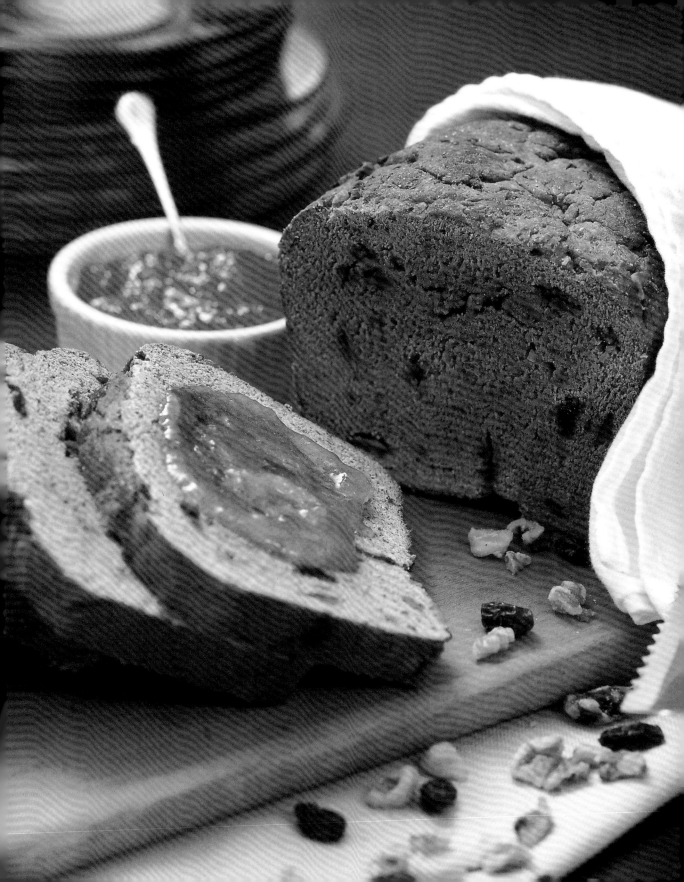

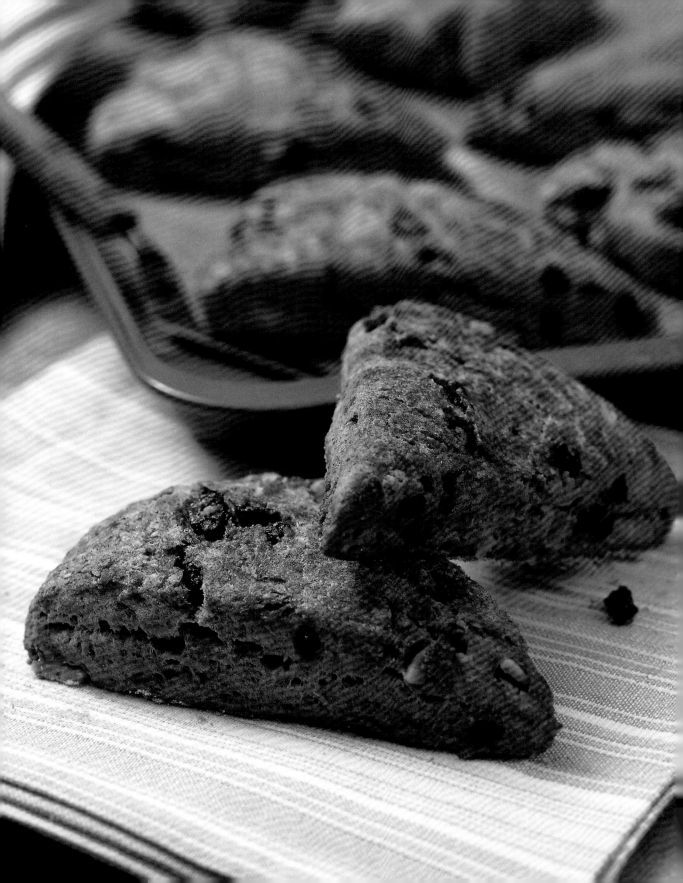

Whole-Wheat Scones
with Dried Cherries and Walnuts

Cherries contain a powerful antioxidant called anthocyanin, which some research has shown to be protective against cancer and inflammation. It is the same pigment that is found in red cabbage and blueberries.

---

2 cups (240 g) whole-wheat flour

1 cup (120 g) all-purpose flour

2 tablespoons (3 g) sugar substitute

½ teaspoon salt

2½ teaspoons baking soda

¾ cup (225 g) omega-3-rich margarine

3 egg whites, divided

1½ tablespoons (20 ml) nonfat milk

1⅓ tablespoons (19 ml) canola oil

¾ cup (185 g) plain nonfat yogurt

¼ cup (30 g) dried cherries, chopped

¼ cup (30 g) walnuts, chopped

Preheat oven to 400°F (200°C, or gas mark 6).

In a large bowl, combine the flours, sugar substitute, salt, and baking soda. Add the margarine and blend with a fork until the mixture forms large crumbs.

In a small bowl, whisk together 2 egg whites, nonfat milk, and canola oil until well blended. Add the yogurt and mix well. Mix into the dry ingredients until just moistened. Stir in the dried cherries and walnuts.

Roll the dough out on a floured surface to about ¾-inch (2-cm) thick. Cut circles or triangles and place each scone on a baking sheet lined with parchment paper. Whisk the remaining egg white and brush over the scones.

Bake 12 to 15 minutes, until tops are golden.

Yield: About 15 scones

Nutritional Analysis: *Each scone provides 200 calories; 12 g fat; 5 g protein; 18 g net carbohydrate; 3 g dietary fiber; and 0 mg cholesterol.*

High-Protein Soy Bread

If you are pressed for time, this recipe works just as well with
a standard breadmaking machine. The wheat gluten called for in this
recipe can be found in the baking section of most grocery stores.

1½ cups (355 ml) warm water (slightly
warmer than body temperature)

1 tablespoon (12 g) dry yeast (1 packet)

2 teaspoons sugar

1 teaspoon salt

2 tablespoons (28 ml) canola oil

⅓ cup (80 ml) soy milk

1½ cups (180 g) soy flour

2 tablespoons (12 g) wheat gluten

½ cup (60 g) flaxseed, ground finely

2½ cups (300 g) whole-wheat flour

½ cup (60 g) walnuts, finely chopped,
optional

Canola oil spray

Place the warm water in a large bowl. Stir in yeast and sugar until dissolved, and let stand until the mixture foams, 5 to 10 minutes. Add salt, canola oil, soy milk, and soy flour. Blend well. Stir in the gluten, flaxseed, and whole-wheat flour, adding the wheat flour last, 1/2 cup (60 g) at a time, until the dough is soft and workable. (Set aside any leftover flour to flour your kneading surface.) Add walnuts, if desired.

Place dough onto a lightly floured surface and knead until smooth and elastic, 8 to 10 minutes. Form dough into a ball. Lightly spray a large bowl with canola oil spray, and place the dough ball in the bowl. Turn the dough once so that the top is lightly coated with oil. Cover with a damp cloth and let rise in a warm place until doubled in volume, about an hour.

Lightly spray a 5 × 9-inch (13 × 22.5-cm) loaf pan with canola spray. Punch down the dough and remove from the bowl. Form into a loaf, tucking the ends under, and place into the loaf pan. If you prefer a crustier product, form into a round loaf, tucking all edges under, and place on a pizza stone instead of in a loaf pan. Cover and let rise once again, until doubled in size (about an hour).

Preheat oven to 375°F (190°C, or gas mark 5). Carefully transfer the loaf pan into the oven, placing it on the center rack. Bake 35 to 40 minutes, or until the top is golden brown and the bottom of the loaf sounds hollow when tapped. Remove and cool on a wire rack.

Yield: 1 loaf (about 12 servings)

Nutritional Analysis: Each slice provides 240 calories; 11 g fat; 12 g protein; 19 g net carbohydrate; 7 g dietary fiber; and 0 mg cholesterol.

Pecan Date Bread with Currants

The new dietary guidelines released by the U.S. Department of Agriculture recommend eating 3 to 5 servings of nuts, seeds, or legumes every day. Pecans are a good source of monounsaturated fats, fiber, and antioxidants. Currants are a great source of vitamin A and iron.

1 cup (150 g) pitted dates, chopped

½ cup (75 g) dried currants

¾ cup (175 ml) boiling water

1 egg white

2¼ (12 ml) teaspoons nonfat milk

2 teaspoons (10 ml) canola oil

½ cup (12 g) sugar substitute

¼ cup (55 g) omega-3-rich margarine

½ cup (60 g) whole-wheat flour

½ cup (60 g) all-purpose flour

⅓ cup (40 g) flaxseed, ground

2 teaspoons baking powder

½ teaspoon salt

¾ teaspoon nutmeg

½ cup (50 g) pecans, chopped

2 tablespoons (8 g) orange zest

Preheat oven to 350°F (180°C, or gas mark 4).

Place dates and currants in a bowl and add boiling water. Set aside. Line the bottom and sides of a loaf pan with parchment paper.

In a medium-size bowl, whisk together the egg white, nonfat milk, and canola oil. Add the sugar substitute and margarine. Beat with an electric mixer until creamy. Stir in the date mixture.

In a large bowl, mix together the flours, flaxseed, baking powder, salt, and nutmeg. Fold in the egg white mixture until just moistened. Fold in the pecans and orange zest.

Pour the batter into the loaf pan and bake 45 to 50 minutes. Let cool in the pan for 10 minutes, transfer to a cooling rack, and allow loaf to cool completely before slicing.

Yield: 1 loaf (about 12 servings or slices)

Nutritional Analysis: Each serving provides 190 calories; 10 g fat; 3 g protein; 21 g net carbohydrate; 4 g dietary fiber; and 0 mg cholesterol.

CHAPTER 4

Change the Energy Imbalance

The problem of excess body weight has received a great deal of attention, and for good reason. Statistics indicate that 65 percent of the U.S. population is burdened with being overweight or obese.

One reason for this growing problem is the increasing imbalance between the amount of calories we consume and those we expend. Calories are a way of measuring energy, so you can think of this balance in the same way you think of your bank account. If you withdraw more than you deposit, your bank balance will go down, and vice versa. Americans' lifestyles have grown increasingly sedentary, starting with the introduction of television, then computers and video games. At the same time, Americans are consuming more calories than in the past. Between 1971 and 2000, the average caloric intake for American women went up by 22 percent (from 1,542 calories to 1,877 calories per day). The average caloric intake for men increased 7 percent during that time (from 2,450 calories to 2,618 calories per day). The "super-size" portion has definitely played a role in this caloric increase. Portion sizes for many commercial foods are bigger than ever.

Energy Balance

Energy balance is a key factor in weight gain and loss. Consuming as little as 12 calories per day in excess of what the body expends for energy can cause a gain of one pound of fat per year. Over the years, this adds up. While our grandparents went out to play or even work in the fields when they were young, today's young people spend much of their time sitting down. This shift in activity level has been a major contributor to the problem of excess weight, which in turn is a risk factor for inflammation.

PHYSICAL ACTIVITY

The best way to address this imbalance is to increase physical activity, while at the same time modifying energy intake (calories). Physical activity is a vital component in this effort because it not only burns excess calories, but it also changes body composition. By engaging in physical activity, our bodies build muscle to meet the needs of that activity. Muscle is a more metabolically active tissue than fat, so increasing the percentage of muscle in the body will burn more calories even when you are at rest. Physical activity has other benefits as well. It raises the level of high-density lipoprotein (HDL), the "good cholesterol" in the blood, strengthens the heart muscles by giving them a good workout, and helps maintain a healthy blood pressure.

REDUCING CALORIES

Modifying the energy content of your diet can be done by taking a careful look at what is in your cupboards, how you shop for groceries, and how you prepare food. When working to reduce calories, I recommend the following:

Do a complete inventory of your kitchen. Read labels for calorie and fat content, and throw out high-calorie/high-fat items. Make a list of the items you discard, and vow not to purchase them again. After all, they are not contributing to your overall health (even if they bring temporary pleasure, they are detrimental in the long run). If you simply must have a particular item once in a while, go ahead. Just make sure you plan ahead of time for how often and how much of the item you will consume. Otherwise, it will be too tempting to reach for it whenever you have a craving.

When you shop for groceries, try this strategy: Shop primarily around the perimeter of the grocery store, choosing fewer items from the center aisles where the majority of the

FYI
Protein supplements will not increase the size or strength of your muscles. In fact, they may increase the risk of heart disease by causing unhealthy changes in blood lipids. Although these products are available in many health food stores, claims made on the product label are not regulated by the Food and Drug Administration. The side effects of these products are still not well known.

processed food products are found. By shopping the perimeter, you will be able to select fresh produce, dairy items, whole-grain breads and products, fresh and frozen fish, and chicken and other lean meats. Processed foods tend to be higher in fat, sugar, and salt, so you'll want to purchase these in moderation.

Take time to read labels and make a list of the healthful items you want to keep on hand in the kitchen. The most important items to note include serving size; calories per serving; and percent total fat, saturated fat, and sodium.

Make sure you note the serving size because this is what all of the rest of the nutrient information is based on. Manufacturers can easily deceive the consumer with unrealistically low serving sizes, which make the product appear more healthful than it really is when a normal serving is consumed. In addition to the calorie content, assess the percent daily value of the total fat, saturated fat, and sodium. Percent daily values are based on a diet of 2,000 calories per day. Using this standard, consumers can assess whether the product is relatively high, medium, or low in a specific nutrient. Items with less than 5 to 10 percent of the daily value are considered to be low in that item, so choose products with fat, saturated fat, and sodium within this range whenever possible. Because caloric needs vary according to age, gender, activity level, and a number of other factors, this guideline does not apply to everyone. For those who need significantly more or less than 2,000 calories per day, the values can be calculated with the information provided about the product. To get a good estimate of your individual diet recommendations, select the "My Pyramid Plan" link on the USDA website found at www.mypyramid.gov, then enter your information and follow the indications given.

Learn to cook with alternate methods that help to reduce calories and fat in your recipes. For example, applesauce makes a great substitute for oil in any cake or cookie recipe. Puréed prunes (easily found in the baby food aisle) make a good substitute for oil in chocolate items such as brownies and chocolate cake. Use cooking oil spray instead of oil or margarine when coating pans for baking or sautéing. Learn to use sugar substitutes in place of sugar, and avoid deep-frying.

These are just a few suggestions for ways you can reduce the calories in the foods you eat. The key is to seek out and put into practice information that will help you develop new patterns for purchasing, preparing, and consuming foods.

FYI
Eating out can threaten your plan to reduce calories in your daily diet. When eating out, choose restaurants that offer healthier foods, salads, and smaller portions. And don't be shy to ask restaurant personnel for information about the food on the menu.

Citrus Pecan Chicken Salad

Clementines are the smallest variety of mandarin oranges.
They are easy to peel, usually seedless, and sweet tasting.
Clementines are best stored in the refrigerator, where they will keep
for 3 to 4 weeks. A single clementine has only about 35 calories, so they
make a great snack, full of vitamins A and C, folate, and lots of fiber.
Pineapple can be substituted for the clementines in this recipe if you'd prefer.

---

5 tablespoons (70 ml) extra virgin olive oil, divided

2 pounds (1 kg) boneless, skinless chicken breast, cubed

¾ cup (175 ml) light, plain soy milk

⅓ teaspoon mustard

3 teaspoons lemon juice

¼ teaspoon salt

¼ teaspoon paprika

3 cups (600 g) seedless clementines, cut into ¾-inch (2-cm) pieces

2 kiwifruit, peeled and cut into ¾-inch (2-cm) pieces

1 cup (100 g) pecans, coarsely chopped

½ cup (50 g) pecan halves, lightly toasted

Salt and pepper to taste

4 cups (120 g) fresh spinach leaves, washed and stemmed

Heat 2 tablespoons (28 ml) of the olive oil over medium-high heat in a large skillet. Add chicken breast and sauté, stirring constantly, until chicken pieces are cooked through. Remove from heat and place in a large bowl. Cover with plastic wrap and chill 1 to 2 hours.

In a blender or food processor, combine soy milk, mustard, lemon juice, salt, and paprika. Process on a low setting, adding in the remaining olive oil a little at a time, so that the mixture thickens and becomes smooth.

Remove chicken from the refrigerator. Add soy milk dressing mixture to chicken and mix well. Gently blend in the clementine, kiwifruit, and pecans. Add salt and pepper to taste.

Serve over spinach leaves and garnish with pecan halves.

Yield: 8 to 10 servings

Nutritional Analysis: Each serving provides 420 calories; 26 g fat; 34 g protein; 12 g net carbohydrate; 4 g dietary fiber; and 86 mg cholesterol.

Baked Sweet Potato Fries

Sweet potatoes are high in fiber, vitamin A, and potassium.

2 sweet potatoes, peeled

3 tablespoons (40 ml) orange juice

Canola oil spray

Salt to taste

Preheat oven to 425°F (220°C, or gas mark 7). Cut sweet potatoes into sticks, about ¼-inch (6-mm) wide. Sprinkle with orange juice, and place on a baking sheet lined with parchment paper. Spray liberally with canola oil spray. Bake for 15 minutes on the middle rack of the oven. Turn the fries, spray again with canola oil spray, and return to the oven. Bake an additional 15 to 20 minutes or until crisp.

Yield: 4 servings

Nutritional Analysis: Each serving provides 60 calories; 1 g fat; 1 g protein; 11 g net carbohydrate; 7 g dietary fiber; and 0 mg cholesterol.

Chilled Yogurt Soup

Yogurt is a great source of calcium and vitamin B12.

One 14-ounce (390 g) can
98 percent fat-free chicken broth

One 32-ounce (905 g) container plain, nonfat yogurt

One 14-ounce (390 g) can tomato purée

1 English cucumber, finely diced

¼ teaspoon ground cumin

¼ cup (25 g) finely chopped mint leaves

In a bowl, combine broth, yogurt, and tomato purée. Stir in cucumber and cumin. Cover and refrigerate 2 to 3 hours, until well chilled. Sprinkle with mint leaves prior to serving.

Yield: 6 to 8 servings

Nutritional Analysis: Each serving provides 94 calories; 0 g fat; 8 g protein; 17 g net carbohydrate; 2 g dietary fiber; and 3 mg cholesterol.

Colorful Low-Cal Coleslaw

Yellow squash are easy to julienne. For this recipe, leave the skin on and trim both ends. Cut the squash in half and lay both halves, cut side down, on a cutting board. Slice into strips about ¼-inch (6-mm) thick. Lay these strips flat and slice into matchsticks ¼-inch (6-mm) thick and 1½-inches (3.75-cm) long. Yellow squash are a good source of vitamins A and C, folate, several minerals, and fiber.

---

1 small red cabbage, cored and shredded

1 yellow squash, julienned

1 carrot, finely shredded

¼ cup (60 ml) lemon juice

½ cup (120 ml) apple cider vinegar

⅓ cup (80 ml) flaxseed oil

⅓ cup (80 ml) canola oil

½ cup (12 g) sugar substitute

2 teaspoons dry mustard

Salt and pepper to taste

Place cabbage, squash, and carrot in a large bowl. In a separate bowl, whisk together the remaining ingredients, adding salt and pepper to taste. Pour over cabbage mixture and toss well. Chill in the refrigerator 3 to 4 hours before serving.

Yield: 10 to 12 servings

Nutritional Analysis: Each serving provides 150 calories; 13 g fat; 1 g protein; 13 g net carbohydrate; 1 g dietary fiber; and 0 mg cholesterol.

FYI

When eating out, ask for salad dressings and mayonnaise on the side and use minimal amounts to reduce your caloric intake. Order items that have been baked, grilled, or steamed, instead of deep-fried or stir-fried. For a more modest meal, order a salad and appetizer instead of a full meal.

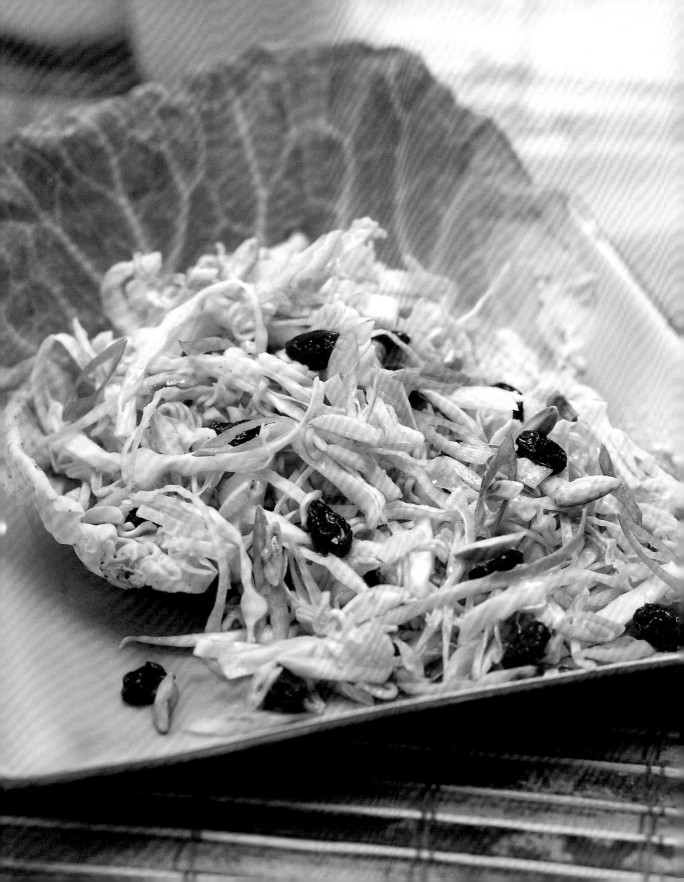

Asian Almond Salad

Almonds are a great source of the antioxidant vitamin E, which is contained in the meat portion of the nut. The almond skins are also important as they contain up to 20 flavonoids. Research indicates that the vitamin E works together with the flavonoids in the skins to nearly double the antioxidant capacity of almonds.

For the dressing:

½ cup (120 ml) almond oil

⅓ cup (80 ml) apple cider vinegar

¼ cup (6 g) sugar substitute

3 tablespoons (40 ml) soy sauce

For the salad:

1 cup (125 g) slivered almonds

One 3-ounce (85 g) package ramen noodles

½ head white cabbage, cored and finely shredded

½ head radicchio, cored and finely shredded

¼ cup (40 g) seedless raisins

2 cups (470 ml) canned mandarin oranges, packed in juice, drained

2 scallions, finely sliced

Combine dressing ingredients in a blender and blend until smooth. Put in refrigerator to chill.

Heat a skillet over medium heat and toast almond slivers, stirring constantly, until they are just golden brown. Remove from heat and allow to cool.

Place the ramen noodles in a large bowl and crush them with a soup ladle or wooden spoon (they should be similar in size to fried chow mein noodles). Add shredded cabbage, radicchio, almonds, raisins, mandarin oranges, and scallions. Mix well and serve with dressing.

Yield: 6 servings

Nutritional Analysis: Each serving provides 380 calories; 28 g fat; 8 g protein; 26 g net carbohydrate; 5 g dietary fiber; and 0 mg cholesterol.

Glazed Chicken with Fresh Date Chutney

Dates are high in fiber, contain iron, and are a great source of potassium. One serving of dates (¼ cup [40 g] chopped dates) contains about 3 grams of fiber, and 7 percent of the recommended daily value of potassium. Tamarind paste is available in many grocery stores (in the international foods section) and in Asian markets. It is made from the pulp of the tamarind fruit, which has a tangy sweet-sour taste and is dark brown in color when mature. Tamarind paste contains vitamin C, which helps your body absorb the iron from the dates.

For the chutney:
½ cup (80 g) golden raisins
1 cup (150 g) dates, pitted and finely chopped
½ cup (120 ml) water
1 teaspoon fresh ginger, minced
1 teaspoon grated orange zest
2 tablespoons (30 g) tamarind paste, optional

1 tablespoon (6 g) cayenne pepper, optional

For the marinade:
⅔ cup (75 ml) orange juice
1 tablespoon (14 ml) soy sauce
1 tablespoon (8 g) cornstarch

Six 4-ounce (115 g) boneless, skinless chicken breast halves, scored

In a medium-size bowl, mix the chutney ingredients. Cover and set aside.

In a small bowl, mix together the orange juice, soy sauce, and cornstarch. Place the chicken in a large bowl and pour in the marinade. Cover the bowl with plastic wrap and refrigerate 30 to 60 minutes.

Preheat broiler. Line a baking pan with parchment paper. Remove the chicken breasts from the marinade, reserving the marinade for basting. Place the chicken breasts in the lined baking pan. Place the pan under the broiler, about 6 inches (15 cm) from the heat. Broil 10 to 15 minutes on each side, basting often with the reserved marinade. Juices should run clear when meat is pierced with a knife. Serve hot with chutney.

Yield: 6 servings

Nutritional Analysis: Each serving provides 275 calories; 3 g fat; 25 g protein; 35 g net carbohydrate; 3 g dietary fiber; and 63 mg cholesterol.

Fiesta Gazpacho with Grilled Shrimp

When my husband, Bryan, added grilled shrimp to gazpacho, a favorite summer dish of ours, he lent a new twist to a great classic! Use locally grown tomatoes for the sweetest taste. This cold soup can be made a day or two ahead as it keeps very well in the refrigerator. Serve with garlic toast or crackers.

---

2 fresh, large tomatoes

1 English cucumber (or 2 regular cucumbers, seeded)

¾ cup (45 g) fresh parsley

1 clove garlic, finely minced

¾ cup (175 ml) red wine vinegar

½ cup (120 ml) canola oil or flaxseed oil

One 48-ounce (1.4-L) can tomato juice, chilled

2 cobs sweet corn, boiled, kernels removed

Salt to taste

2 pounds (1 kg) raw shrimp, peeled and deveined, with tails left on

1 teaspoon seafood seasoning, optional

Canola oil spray

1 fresh lime

Finely chop tomatoes, cucumbers, and parsley (saving 8 sprigs for garnish). Place in a large mixing bowl. Add garlic, vinegar, oil, tomato juice, corn kernels, and salt to taste. Mix well. If you prefer a puréed consistency, place mixture in food processor and blend until smooth. Put gazpacho in refrigerator to chill for 2 to 3 hours.

Just prior to serving, rinse raw shrimp in cold water. Spray grilling surface with canola oil and place shrimp on grill. Cook shrimp 2 to 3 minutes on each side, sprinkling with seafood seasoning as desired.

Ladle gazpacho into individual serving bowls. Place shrimp in the center of each bowl, on top of the gazpacho. Garnish with parsley and a lime wedge.

Yield: 8 servings

Nutritional Analysis: Each serving provides 382 calories; 21 g fat; 31 g protein; 17 g net carbohydrate; 3 g dietary fiber; and 209 mg cholesterol.

(pictured on next page)

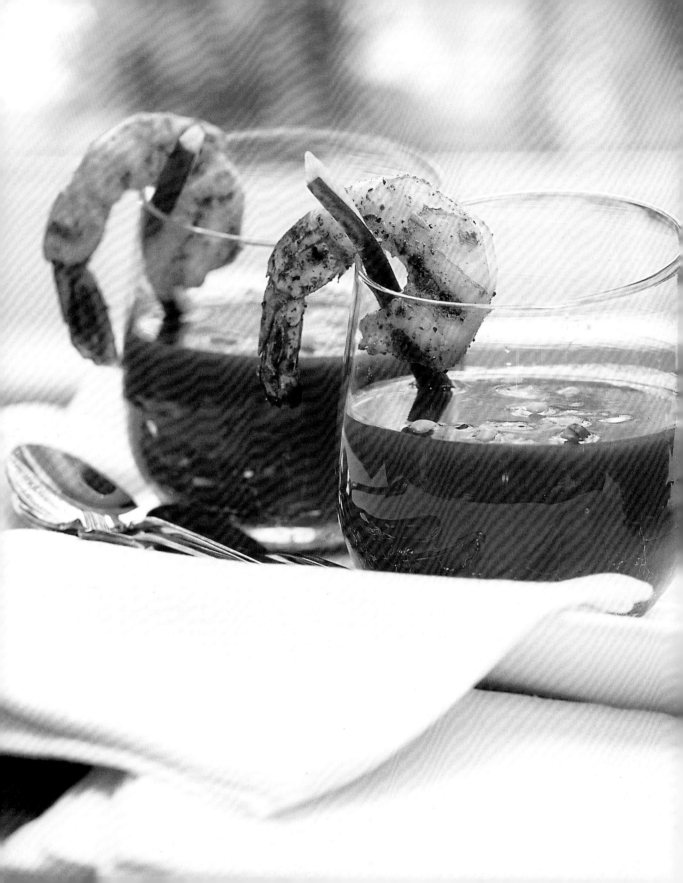

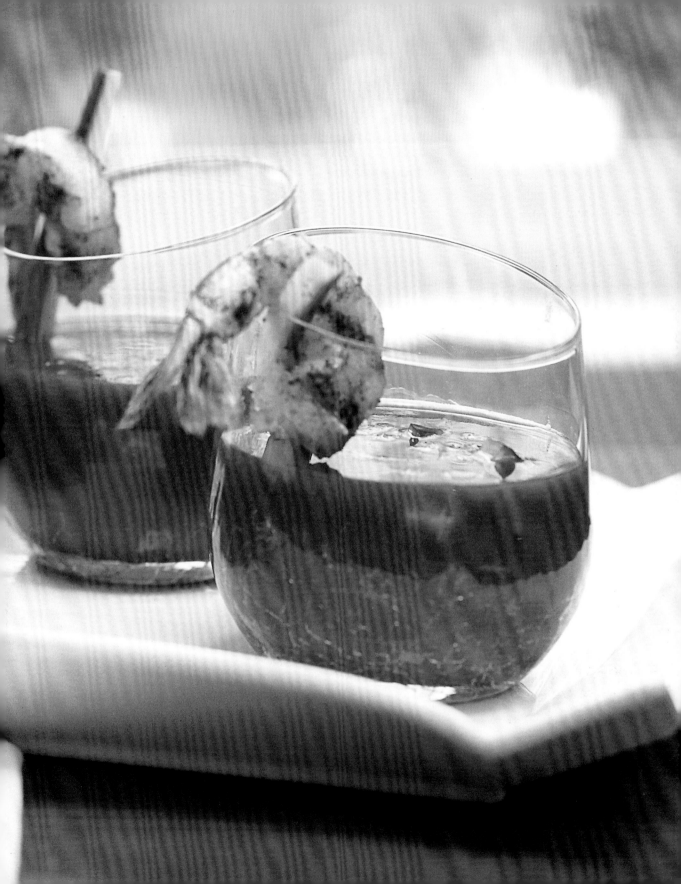

Flaxseed Crackers
with Roasted Red Pepper Hummus

I make my hummus from scratch so it comes out smooth. I put the beans in a slow cooker on low heat before heading to work, and when I come home, they are ready to go. If you're short on time, or do not have a slow cooker, 2 cans (15 ounces [420 g] each) of chickpeas can be used instead of the dry beans.

For the hummus:

2 cups (500 g) dry chickpeas

1 teaspoon garlic, minced

½ teaspoon salt

½ cup (120 g) tahini

½ cup (120 ml) lemon juice

¾ cup (90 g) roasted red peppers, finely chopped

¼ teaspoon dried basil

2 tablespoons (28 ml) extra virgin olive oil

For the crackers:

¾ cup (90 g) all-purpose flour

¼ cup (30 g) flaxseed, ground

4 tablespoons (56 g) omega-3-rich margarine, softened

1 teaspoon Worcestershire sauce

1 teaspoon seafood seasoning, optional

Pinch of salt

For the appetizers:

1 English cucumber, sliced

½ pint (175 g) cherry tomatoes, halved

To make the hummus: Place the dry garbanzo beans in a medium-size slow cooker, and add 4 to 5 cups (1 L to 1.2 L) of water. Mix in the minced garlic. Cook on low until soft, 8 to 10 hours. Drain the beans and put in a food processor or blender, along with the remaining ingredients for the hummus. Process until smooth. Put in serving dish, cover and chill until ready to serve.

To make the crackers: In a medium-size mixing bowl, blend the flour, flaxseed, and margarine until the mixture forms large clumps. Add remaining ingredients, and mix well. Form into a roll about 1½ inches (3.75 cm) in diameter. Wrap and chill for 2 hours.

Preheat oven to 425°F (220°C, or gas mark 7). Remove cracker dough from refrigerator and slice into rounds ¼-inch (6-mm) thick. Carefully place on baking sheets lined with parchment paper, and flatten each cracker with the side of a large butcher's knife or rolling pin to make thinner. Bake 10 to 12 minutes, or until rounds are slightly brown around the edges. Remove from oven and slide the parchment paper onto a cooling rack, taking care not to break the rounds. Cool for 5 to 6 minutes.

Prior to serving, remove hummus from refrigerator.

To make the appetizers: Top each cracker with a small spoonful of hummus, and a cucumber round or cherry tomato half.

Yield: 25 to 30 appetizers

Nutritional Analysis: Each appetizer provides 120 calories; 6 g fat; 4 g protein; 10 g net carbohydrate; 3 g dietary fiber; and 0 mg cholesterol.

Puréed Cauliflower with Parsley

This high-fiber dish is a wonderful alternative to
mashed potatoes and is considerably lower in calories.

---

1 small head cauliflower, cored and
   broken into florets

½ teaspoon salt

2 tablespoons (28 g) omega-3-rich
   margarine

⅛ cup (7.5 g) fresh parsley, finely
   chopped, divided

Place cauliflower florets into a large pot and add 1 to 1½ cups (235 to 355 ml) water. Cover and bring to a boil over medium-high heat. Reduce heat and simmer until cauliflower is tender (8 to 10 minutes). Transfer to a blender or food processor. Add salt, margarine, and half of the parsley, and process on high until cauliflower is smooth and creamy.

Serve topped with remaining chopped parsley.

Yield: 6 servings

Nutritional Analysis: Each serving provides 34 calories; 4 g fat; 0 g protein; 1 g net carbohydrate; 1 g dietary fiber; and 0 mg cholesterol.

Braised Red Cabbage
with Apple and Red Wine

Red cabbage is an excellent source of antioxidant polyphenols that studies suggest may protect brain cells against oxidative stress. Red cabbage also provides six to eight times more vitamin C than white cabbage, and it is more flavorful. Avoid precut cabbage because cabbage begins to lose its valuable vitamin C content as soon as it is cut. Red cabbage will keep nicely in a plastic bag in your refrigerator for about two weeks. The alcohol from the wine in this recipe will evaporate during cooking, but you will still enjoy the benefit of the flavonoids it contains.

---

1 small head of red cabbage

3 red apples, thinly sliced

¼ cup (40 g) dried currants

1 teaspoon sugar substitute

¼ teaspoon ground cinnamon

¼ teaspoon ground nutmeg

¼ teaspoon ground cloves

Salt and pepper to taste

Canola oil spray

¼ cup (60 ml) dry red wine

¼ cup (60 ml) cider vinegar

Preheat oven to 300°F (150°C, or gas mark 2).

Discard the outer leaves of the cabbage, cut into quarters, and remove the core. Shred the cabbage with a sharp knife. In a large bowl, mix apple slices, currants, sugar substitute, and spices. Spray a large casserole dish with canola oil spray, and layer the shredded cabbage and apple mixture alternately, until both are used up. Mix together the redwine and cider vinegar, and pour over the apple-cabbage mixture.

Place casserole dish in the oven with a tight lid, and bake 45 to 60 minutes, stirring once or twice, until cabbage is tender.

Yield: 8 to 10 servings

Nutritional Analysis: Each serving provides 95 calories; 4 g fat; 1 g protein; 15 g net carbohydrate; 3 g dietary fiber; and 0 mg cholesterol.

FYI
In addition to antioxidant protection, apples provide both soluble and insoluble fiber, which help to lower cholesterol. The soluble fiber in apples, called pectin, can also remove such toxins from the body as lead and mercury.

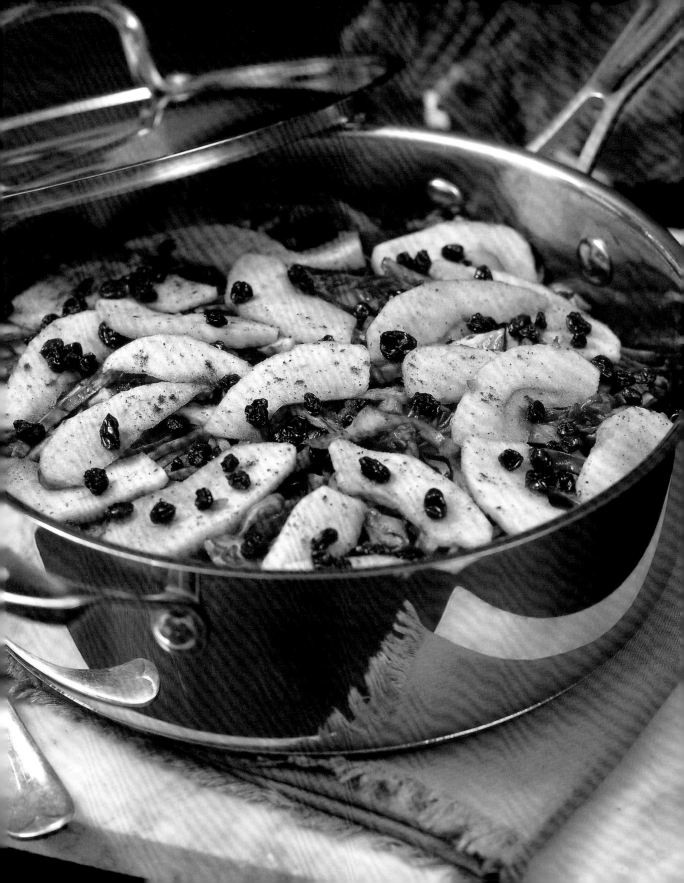

Maryland Crab Soup

My mother-in-law made crab soup often, to the delight of her family. Her boys were set to work picking crabmeat from the crabs while she prepared to make the soup. This version is modified but is every bit as tasty, and saves a lot of time by using lump crabmeat. Because crabmeat is highly perishable, I recommend purchasing it the same day you plan to use it, and do not allow it to stand at room temperature for an extended length of time. Once cooked, it keeps for only 2 to 3 days in the refrigerator.

Two 14-ounce (390 g) cans vegetable broth

1 cup (235 ml) tomato sauce

1 medium onion, diced

2 celery stalks, finely diced

1 tablespoon (4 g) fresh thyme, finely chopped

1 bay leaf

2 tablespoons (18 g) seafood seasoning

½ cup (92 g) barley

1 pound (455 g) lump crabmeat

2 cups (140 g) shredded green cabbage

2 carrots, finely diced

1 large potato, diced

Salt and pepper to taste

Place the first 9 ingredients in a large soup pot. Bring to a boil, reduce heat, and simmer 40 to 50 minutes on low heat. Add vegetables and cook for another 20 to 25 minutes, until potatoes are tender.

Yield: 4 to 6 servings

Nutritional Analysis: *Each serving provides 240 calories; 2 g fat; 23 g protein; 30 g net carbohydrate; 6 g dietary fiber; and 64 mg cholesterol.*

Grilled Catfish Sandwich

Catfish is one of the more lean types of fish, with approximately 210 calories per a 6-ounce (170 g) serving. For this recipe, you'll want to purchase fresh fish fillets, with no drying or browning around the edges. Use the fillets within two days of purchase, and cook to an internal temperature of 145°F (65°C).

Four 6-ounce (170 g) catfish fillets

¼ cup (35 g) cornmeal

2 teaspoons cumin

1 teaspoon salt

½ teaspoon cayenne pepper, optional

2 egg whites, beaten

Canola oil spray

4 whole-wheat sandwich buns

4 to 8 leaves red leaf lettuce

1 tomato, sliced

Dijon mustard to taste

Rinse catfish fillets and pat dry with a paper towel. Place cornmeal, cumin, salt, and cayenne pepper in a shallow dish and mix well. Place egg whites in a separate shallow dish. Dredge catfish fillets first in egg whites, then in cornmeal mixture, pressing in cornmeal to coat the fillets well. Spray both sides of each fillet with canola oil spray.

Grill fillets 3 to 4 minutes per side, on a grill set for 375°F to 400°F (190°C to 200°C) with the lid on. Serve with whole wheat sandwich buns, lettuce, tomato, and Dijon mustard.

Yield: 4 servings

Nutritional Analysis: Each serving provides 450 calories; 19 g fat; 40 g protein; 26 g net carbohydrate; 4 g dietary fiber; and 100 mg cholesterol.

FYI

Large-portion sizes have contributed greatly to the obesity epidemic. Throughout the food and restaurant industry, larger-than-ever portions are being served in an effort to attract consumers. The results of "super-sizing" are evident in the increase in Americans' average body weight, to the detriment of our health.

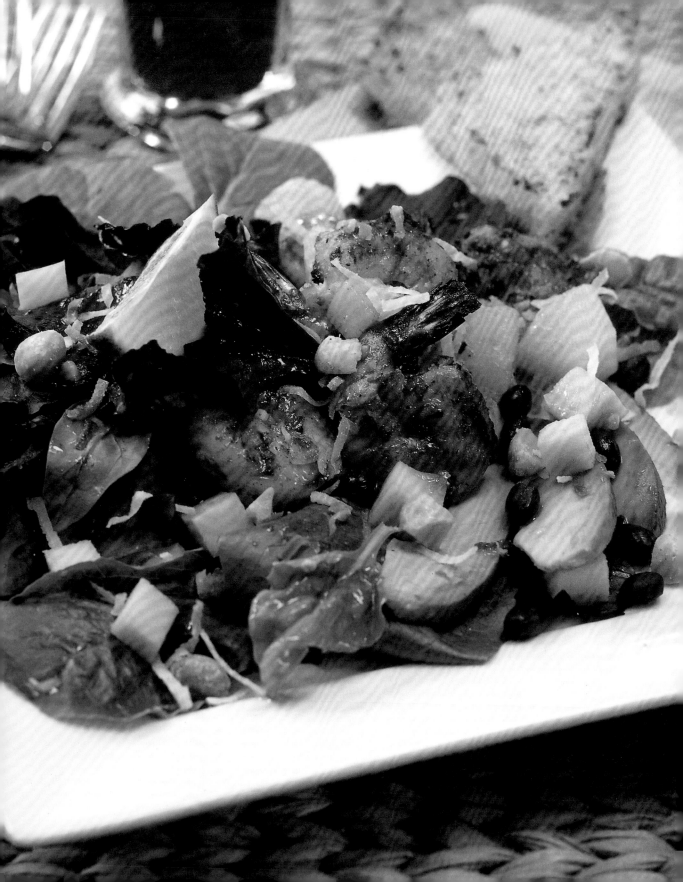

Grilled Shrimp Salad with Macadamia Nuts and Pomegranate Dressing

Shrimp are high in protein and very low in fat.

For the dressing:

½ teaspoon Dijon mustard

¼ cup (60 ml) pomegranate juice

¼ cup (60 ml) lemon juice

¼ cup (60 ml) walnut oil

Salt and pepper to taste

For the salad:

1 pound (455 g) large shrimp, peeled and deveined

2 tablespoons (28 ml) extra virgin olive oil

2 teaspoons lemon zest

1 teaspoon garlic, finely minced

1 avocado, peeled and sliced thinly

2 mangos, peeled and cut into 1-inch (2.5-cm) cubes

One 8-ounce (225 g) can pineapple chunks, packed in unsweetened juice

1 teaspoon lime juice

⅓ cup (40 g) macadamia nuts

½ cup (45 g) sweetened coconut

8 cups (160 g) mixed spring greens

One 15-ounce (420 g) can black beans, rinsed and drained

To make the dressing: Place dressing ingredients in a jar with an airtight lid, and shake vigorously. Chill in the refrigerator 30 to 40 minutes.

To make the salad: Toss shrimp in a bowl with olive oil, lemon zest, and garlic. Cover and place in refrigerator for 45 minutes. Place avocado, mango, and pineapple chunks in a large mixing bowl, and toss gently with lime juice. Spread macadamia nuts in a baking pan, and position pan in the oven on the middle rack. Toast under the broiler 3 to 4 minutes, stirring often, until toasted. Cool and chop into large pieces. Lightly toast coconut under broiler, stirring often. Heat grill and grill shrimp 2 to 2½ minutes on each side, until they appear opaque.

Divide the mixed spring greens between 6 salad plates. Sprinkle black beans over each salad, and top with the avocado-fruit mixture. Place the shrimp on top, sprinkle each salad with macadamia nuts and toasted coconut, and drizzle with dressing.

Yield: 6 servings

Nutritional Analysis: Each serving provides 465 calories; 28 g fat; 22 g protein; 33 g net carbohydrate; 10 g dietary fiber; and 147 mg cholesterol.

Black Bean Burritos
with Avocado and Mango

Cooking beans from scratch is a cinch with a slow cooker. The key is to place the beans in a cooker (2 cups [430 g] dry will yield 4 cups [860 g] cooked), cover with twice as much water, and add one or two crushed cloves of garlic (but not the salt). Adding salt before they are cooked will make the beans less tender.

---

3 tablespoons (40 ml) canola oil

1 small red onion, finely chopped

1 tablespoon (10 g) garlic, minced

2 teaspoons jalapeno peppers, minced

4 cups (400 g) black beans,
  cooked and drained

¼ cup (15 g) fresh cilantro, finely chopped

1 mango, diced

1 avocado, diced

2 teaspoons lime juice

4 large whole-wheat tortillas

Low-fat sour cream, optional

Heat canola oil over medium heat. Add red onion, garlic, and jalapeno peppers, and sauté 1 to 2 minutes, stirring constantly. Add beans and sauté 3 to 4 minutes.

In a medium-size bowl, mix together the cilantro, mango, avocado, and lime juice.

Heat tortillas in the oven or in a dry skillet on top of the stove. Place on individual serving dishes, topped first with the bean mixture, followed by the mango-avocado mixture.

Serve with low-fat sour cream, if desired.

Yield: 4 servings

Nutritional Analysis: Each serving provides 480 calories; 19 g fat; 18 g protein; 45 g net carbohydrate; 21 g dietary fiber; and 0 mg cholesterol.

Orange Mango Chicken Fajitas

To make this dish even more colorful, add one orange bell pepper
to the mix. Bell peppers contain valuable flavonoids,
known for their antioxidant activity, so the more the better!

⅔ cup (75 ml) freshly squeezed orange juice

1 fresh jalapeno pepper, stemmed, seeded, and chopped

1 tablespoon (10 g) garlic, finely chopped

1 teaspoon salt

½ cup (30 g) fresh cilantro, chopped (set aside 4 sprigs for garnish)

1 tablespoon (14 ml) lime juice

Four 4-ounce (115 g) boneless, skinless chicken breasts, cut into strips

2 tablespoons (28 ml) olive oil

1 red onion, sliced

½ teaspoon paprika

½ teaspoon cumin

1 teaspoon dried chile pepper, optional

1 red bell pepper, seeded, cored, and sliced

1 green bell pepper, seeded, cored, and sliced

1 mango, semi-firm, peeled and sliced into strips

Lemon pepper to taste

4 large whole-grain tortillas

Mango or orange slices for garnish

In a large bowl, mix together the orange juice, jalapeno pepper, garlic, salt, cilantro, and lime juice. Add chicken strips, mixing to coat all of the strips, and place in the refrigerator for 1 to 2 hours.

Remove chicken from refrigerator and drain off marinade. Place olive oil in a large frying pan over medium-high heat. Once the oil is fairly hot, sauté the chicken strips and onion until the chicken is cooked through. Add paprika, cumin, and dried chile pepper, stirring until chicken is evenly coated with the spices. Add the bell peppers and mango, and stir-fry for another 3 to 5 minutes, until the peppers are just tender. Season with lemon pepper to taste.

Warm the tortillas in the oven, directly on the rack under the broiler, for 30 to 60 seconds, turning once. Serve the fajita mix wrapped in the tortillas and garnish with a sprig of cilantro and a slice of mango or orange.

Yield: 4 servings

Nutritional Analysis: Each serving provides 466 calories; 14 g fat; 36 g protein; 50 g net carbohydrate; 5 g dietary fiber; and 74 mg cholesterol.

(pictured on next page)

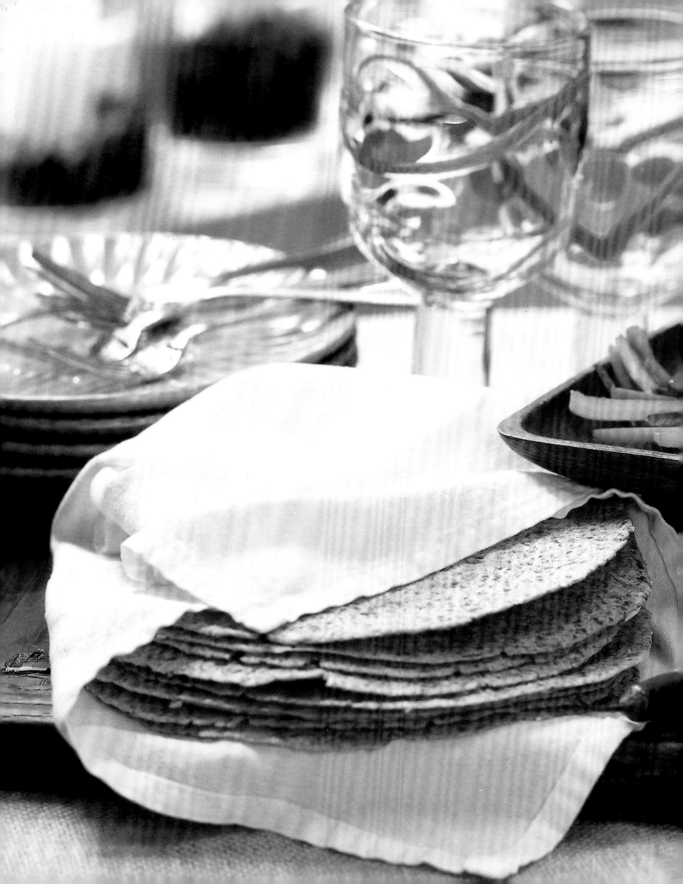

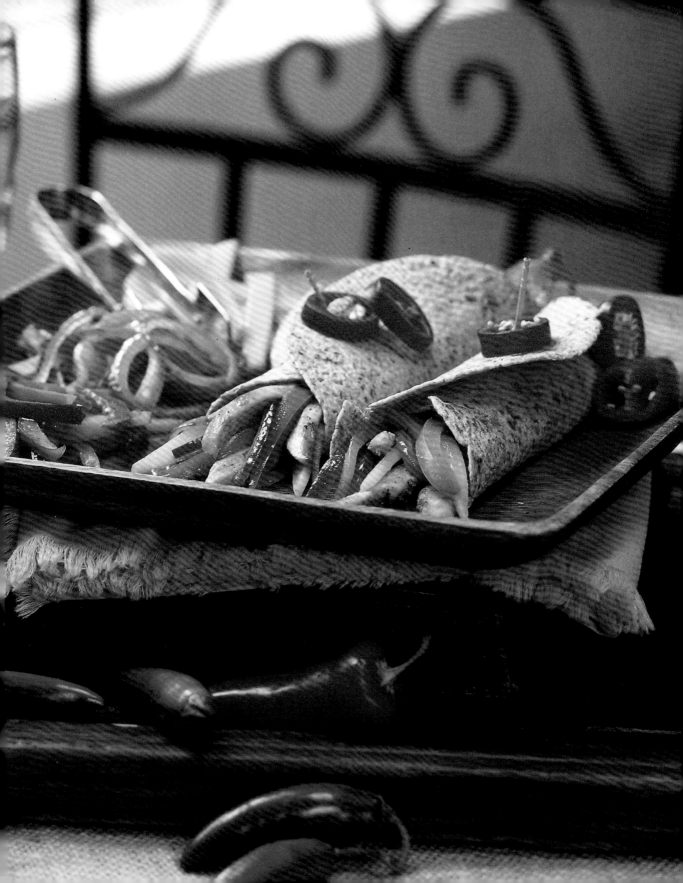

Oven-Baked Chicken Curry with Wild Rice

My mother served this delicious dish often at our house, pleasing family and guests alike. I have adapted it to reduce the calorie and fat content, and find that it is still delicious! Serve with fat-free plain yogurt mixed with chopped cucumber for a well-rounded meal.

One 14½-ounce (405-g) can 98 percent
   fat-free chicken broth, divided

½ cup (80 g) wild rice, uncooked

One 10.75-ounce (301 g) can 98 percent
   fat-free cream of mushroom soup

1 teaspoon ground coriander

½ teaspoon ground cumin

¼ teaspoon turmeric powder

2 teaspoons curry powder

Canola oil spray

Four 4-ounce (115 g) boneless,
   skinless chicken breasts

½ cup (120 ml) water, approximately

½ cup (95 g) brown rice, uncooked

⅓ cup (60 g) almonds, slivered

1 tablespoon (14 ml) extra virgin olive oil

½ cup (50 g) fresh mushrooms, sliced

Salt and pepper

Preheat the oven to 400°F (200°C or gas mark 6).

In a small pot, bring 1¼ cups (295 ml) chicken broth to a boil. Add the wild rice, reduce heat, cover, and simmer for about 1 hour, or until tender.

Mix the mushroom soup and spices in a large bowl until well blended. Spray a shallow baking dish with canola oil. Arrange chicken pieces evenly in the dish. Pour the soup mixture over the chicken. Place on the middle rack of the oven and bake 50 to 55 minutes.

In a separate pot, bring remaining broth and water to a boil. Add the brown rice, reduce heat, cover, and simmer 35 to 40 minutes, or until tender.

Toast the almonds in a dry skillet over medium-high heat until just browned. Remove and set aside.

Heat olive oil in the skillet and add mushrooms. Sauté mushrooms until tender.

Combine the wild rice, brown rice, mushrooms, and almonds in a large bowl. Add salt and pepper to taste. Serve topped with a chicken breast and mushroom sauce.

Yield: 4 servings

Nutritional Analysis: Each serving provides 480 calories; 18 g fat; 36 g protein; 39 g net carbohydrate; 4 g dietary fiber; and 75 mg cholesterol.

Soybean Minestrone Soup

Numerous studies have shown that soy foods are
beneficial in lowering blood-cholesterol levels. Black soybeans
have a more mild taste than other types of soybeans.

---

3 tablespoons (40 ml) extra virgin olive oil

1 large onion, finely chopped

1 leek, finely chopped

2 celery stocks, finely chopped

One 14-ounce (425-ml) can
   vegetable broth

2 carrots, diced

4 red potatoes, diced

2 zucchini, diced

One 14½-ounce (405 g)
   can diced tomatoes

One 15-ounce (420 g) can black soybeans

1 bay leaf

1 tablespoon (4 g) fresh oregano,
   finely chopped

1 tablespoon (4 g) fresh basil,
   finely chopped

1 sprig fresh thyme, finely chopped

1 tablespoon (10 g) garlic, minced

1 cup (30 g) fresh spinach,
   washed and chopped

Salt and pepper to taste

In a large skillet, heat the olive oil over medium-high heat. Add onion, leek, and celery, and sauté 3 to 4 minutes.

In a large pot, bring the vegetable broth to a boil, reduce heat, and add the sautéed vegetables. Add the remaining ingredients, except for spinach, and simmer for 20 minutes, until potatoes are soft. Add the spinach and cook 2 to 3 minutes longer.

Yield: 6 to 8 servings

Nutritional Analysis: *Each serving provides 230 calories; 9 g fat; 9 g protein; 25 g net carbohydrate; 7 g dietary fiber; and 0 mg cholesterol.*

FYI
Soybeans are now available in most grocery stores. Canned soybeans are similar to home-cooked beans in terms of nutrient value. Many salad bars now also feature soybeans, and soy nuts make an excellent snack!

Pink Salmon Cakes
with Mango-Raspberry Chutney

This is a quick recipe that works well on a weeknight, when there may
be little time to prepare and cook. Don't worry about leaving the
salmon bones from the canned salmon in the dish—they are so soft
that they blend into other ingredients. Moreover, the edible salmon bones
are a terrific source of calcium, and they don't change the taste of the dish.
Make the chutney ahead of time and store in the refrigerator for up to 5 days.

For the salmon cakes:

3 egg whites

2¼ tablespoons (30 ml) nonfat milk

2 tablespoons (28 ml) olive oil

2 cans pink salmon, drained

1 cup (30 g) fresh spinach, washed and
    finely chopped

⅓ cup (40 g) all-purpose flour

½ teaspoon salt

Canola oil spray

For the chutney:

2 mangoes, semi-firm, chopped into
    small pieces

1 large tomato, chopped

¼ cup (15 g) fresh cilantro, finely chopped

1 pint (300 g) fresh raspberries

½ cup (50 g) sweet corn kernels, cooked

1 tablespoon (14 ml) hot sauce, optional

To make the salmon cakes: Whisk egg whites, nonfat milk, and olive oil together in a medium-size bowl. Place salmon in a large bowl without removing the bones and mash well with a fork. Add spinach, egg white mixture, flour, and salt. Blend well. Mixture should be slightly moist. Form salmon into palm-size cakes, about ¼-inch (6-mm) thick. Heat a skillet on medium-high heat, and spray with canola oil. Place the salmon cakes into the skillet, and cook until golden brown on both sides.

To make the chutney: In a medium-size bowl, mix mangoes, tomato, and fresh cilantro. Gently mix in fresh raspberries, corn, and hot sauce (if desired). Serve with salmon cakes.

Yield: 4 servings

*Nutritional Analysis: Each serving provides 365 calories; 15 g fat; 23 g protein;
31 g net carbohydrate; 8 g dietary fiber; and 54 mg cholesterol.*

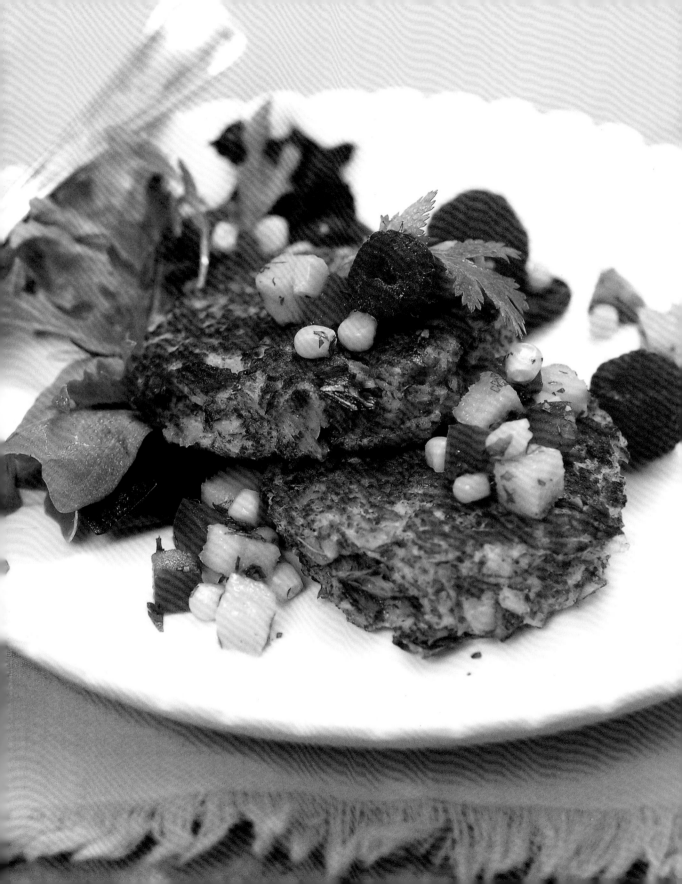

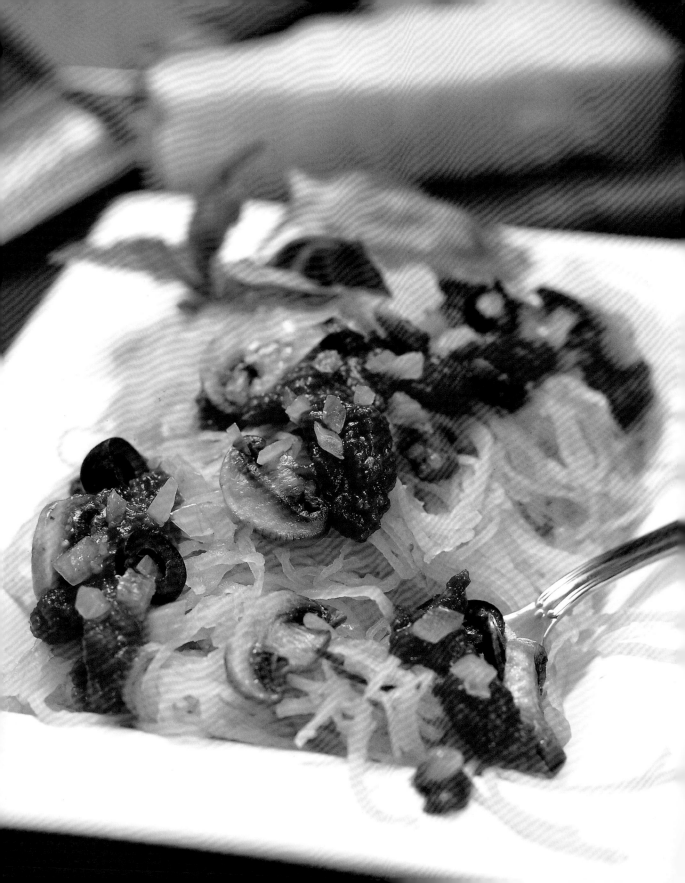

Spaghetti Squash with Bell Pepper Marinara Sauce

In addition to containing flavonoids, basil oil has been proven to restrict bacterial growth.

1 medium-size spaghetti squash

2½ pounds (1.1 kg) sweet red, yellow, and orange peppers

4 teaspoons garlic, finely chopped

¾ cup (175 ml) water

One 6-ounce (170 g) can tomato paste

2 tablespoons (28 ml) extra virgin olive oil

1 small yellow onion, finely diced

1 cup (100 g) fresh mushrooms, sliced

1 cup (100 g) black olives, pitted and sliced

2 medium-size tomatoes, diced

⅓ cup (20 g) fresh basil

2 tablespoons (28 ml) balsamic vinegar

¼ cup (60 ml) dry red wine

Salt and pepper to taste

1 orange, sliced

Preheat oven to 375°F (190°C, or gas mark 5). Slice spaghetti squash in half lengthwise, and scoop out the seeds. Bake the squash, face down, on a cookie sheet lightly sprayed with olive oil spray for about 30 minutes, or until the squash is easily pierced with a fork. Remove from oven and set aside to cool slightly.

Increase oven temperature to 425°F (220°C, or gas mark 7). Core and stem the sweet peppers. Cut into quarters and place peppers, cut side down, on 2 large baking sheets lined with foil. Roast for 20 to 25 minutes, until peppers are tender and tops are browned. Set aside to cool.

Scoop out insides of spaghetti squash, and place in an oven-proof dish. Cover with foil. Reduce oven temperature to 150°F (65°C), and place dish in the oven to keep warm.

In a blender, combine the peppers, garlic, water, and tomato paste. Process until nearly smooth.

Heat olive oil over medium heat. Add onion, mushrooms, and olives, and sauté 4 to 5 minutes, stirring often, until mushrooms are well cooked. Stir in tomatoes, basil, vinegar, and wine, setting aside a few sprigs of basil for the garnish. Cook over low heat until sauce begins to bubble. Season with salt and pepper to taste.

Serve sauce over the spaghetti squash, and garnish with an orange slice and basil sprigs.

Yield: 4 servings

Nutritional Analysis: Each serving provides 280 calories; 10 g fat; 7 g protein; 36 g net carbohydrate; 13 g dietary fiber; and 0 mg cholesterol.

Broiled Mahimahi with Pineapple-Mango Chutney

Although you may not be visiting the islands, this dish will make you feel as if you are! If you don't have fresh pineapple, use canned pineapple packed in unsweetened juice. This dish is great accompanied by mango pecan rice and a side salad.

For the fish:

4 (6-ounce [170 g]) mahimahi fillets

Canola oil spray

2 teaspoons (10 ml) lemon juice

2 teaspoons (10 ml) pineapple juice

2 tablespoons (28 ml) teriyaki sauce

Salt and pepper

For the chutney:

1 cup (200 g) fresh pineapple, chopped

1 mango, peeled and diced

1 kiwi fruit, peeled and diced

1 scallion, sliced very thin

½ sweet red pepper, finely chopped

3 tablespoons (12 g) cilantro, finely chopped

2 teaspoons (10 ml) lime juice

1 teaspoon almond oil or walnut oil

¼ teaspoon salt

⅛ teaspoon crushed red pepper, optional

1 lime, quartered

4 sprigs cilantro for garnishing

Spray mahimahi fillets lightly with canola oil. Place fish on a broiler pan. In a small bowl, blend lemon juice, pineapple juice, and teriyaki sauce, adding salt and pepper to taste, and sprinkle over fish fillets. Broil for 10 to 15 minutes, until fish flakes easily with a fork. Turn off broiler and place fish on a lower rack until ready to serve.

In a small mixing bowl, combine the chutney ingredients. Serve each portion of fish topped with chutney and garnished with a lime wedge and a sprig of cilantro.

Yield: 4 servings

Nutritional Analysis: Each serving provides 290 calories; 4 g fat; 42 g protein; 20 g net carbohydrate; 2 g dietary fiber; and 160 mg cholesterol.

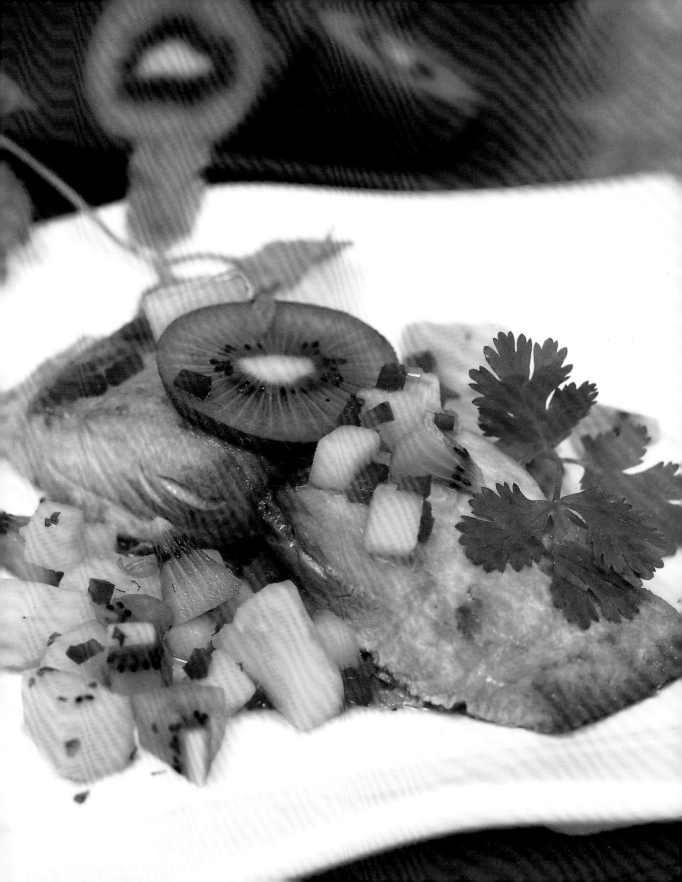

Whole-Wheat Tandoori Chicken Pizza

Pizza dough can be made easily with a standard bread machine. Simply add the dough ingredients to the machine in the order recommended by the manufacturer, set the dough cycle and press "start." After 5 minutes, check the consistency of the dough, and add 1 to 2 tablespoons (14 to 28 ml) of water if needed. When the cycle is complete, the dough is ready to be kneaded.

For the chicken:

1¼ pounds (570 g) skinless, boneless chicken breasts, cut into ½-inch (1-cm) cubes

½ tablespoon (7 ml) lime juice

Salt to taste

1 small onion

1½ teaspoons ground cumin

1½ teaspoons ground coriander

1 teaspoon cayenne pepper

¼ teaspoon ground cardamom

¼ teaspoon ground cinnamon

2 whole cloves

½ teaspoon fresh ginger root, grated

¾ cups (185 g) plain, nonfat yogurt

2 drops red food coloring, optional

For the dough:

1½ teaspoons active dry yeast

¾ cup (175 ml) very warm water (about 110°F [43°C])

1½ cups (180 g) all-purpose flour, divided

¾ cup (90 g) whole-wheat flour

¾ teaspoon kosher salt

1 tablespoon (14 ml) extra virgin olive oil

Olive oil spray

For the topping:

One 8-ounce (225 g) can tomato sauce

¼ cup (15 g) fresh cilantro, finely chopped

To prepare the chicken: Place chicken pieces in a shallow glass or ceramic dish. Sprinkle with lime juice and salt. Set aside. Place the remaining ingredients for the chicken in a blender, and process until smooth. Pour over the chicken and cover. Marinate in the refrigerator 6 to 12 hours.

To make the dough: In a small bowl, whisk together the yeast and warm water. Let stand until foamy, about 5 minutes. In a large bowl, combine 1¼ cups (150 g) of the all-purpose flour, the wheat flour, and salt.

Whisk the olive oil into the yeast mixture. Slowly add the yeast mixture to the flour mixture, stirring with a fork constantly, until the dough forms a slightly sticky ball. Lightly flour a smooth surface with the remaining ¼ cup (30g) flour. Knead the dough on the surface until smooth and elastic, about 10 minutes. Form into a smooth ball.

Spray the inside of a large glass or ceramic bowl with olive oil spray. Place the dough in the bowl, and turn once so that the top side is lightly coated with olive oil. Cover the bowl with a clean, slightly dampened dish towel, and let the dough rise in a warm place until doubled in size, 45 to 60 minutes.

Meanwhile, preheat oven to 400°F (200°C, or gas mark 6). Drain the excess marinade from the chicken pieces, and place the pieces in a roasting pan. Cook 25 to 30 minutes, stirring periodically, until all of the pieces are cooked through. Remove from the oven and set aside.

Increase the oven temperature to 450°F (230°C, or gas mark 8) and preheat a pizza stone for about 30 minutes.

To form the pizza crust: Place the dough ball on a lightly floured surface, and sprinkle a little flour on top. Using your fingertips, flatten the ball to a thick round. Using a rolling pin, roll out the dough until it is about ¼-inch (6-mm) thick, turning and lightly flouring as needed to keep the dough from sticking. Turn the edges of each round to form a slight rim. Spray the surface lightly with olive oil spray.

Carefully slide the dough onto the preheated pizza stone. Spread the tomato sauce evenly over the crust, and sprinkle the chopped cilantro on top. Arrange tandoori chicken pieces over the sauce and herbs. Bake until the crust is golden brown, 8 to 10 minutes. Slice on a cutting board with a pizza knife and serve hot.

Yield: One 12-to 14-inch (30-to 35-cm) pizza (4 servings)

Nutritional Analysis: Each serving provides 470 calories; 8 g fat; 39 g protein; 54 g net carbohydrate; 7 g dietary fiber; and 79 mg cholesterol.

Veggie Burgers

Veggie burgers are made with a wide variety of ingredients. This recipe is a winner for the fiber and antioxidant nutrients it provides. For added protein, mix in 1 cup of puréed, cooked soybeans and add in one more egg white.

---

3 egg whites

2 tablespoons (28 ml) plus 1 teaspoon
  (5 ml) nonfat milk

4 tablespoons (56 ml) olive oil, divided

2 carrots, grated

1 potato, grated

1 zucchini, grated

¼ cup (30 g) onion, finely chopped

½ teaspoon salt

½ teaspoon black pepper

¼ teaspoon ground cumin

6 whole-wheat hamburger buns

Dijon mustard

Lettuce and tomato slices, optional

In a large bowl, whisk together egg whites, nonfat milk, and 2 tablespoons (28 ml) of olive oil. Add carrots, potatoes, zucchini, onion, salt, pepper, and cumin. Mix until the vegetable mixture is well coated.

Heat the remaining 2 tablespoons (28 ml) of olive oil in a large skillet over medium-high heat. Scoop about ½ cup of the vegetable mixture into the skillet for each burger. Fry 3 to 4 minutes on each side, until golden brown. Remove from skillet and place onto paper towels to absorb extra oil. Serve hot on hamburger buns with a dash of Dijon mustard, lettuce, and tomato slices.

Yield: 6 burgers

Nutritional Analysis: Each serving provides 235 calories; 12 g fat; 7 g protein; 23 g net carbohydrate; 6 g dietary fiber; and 0 mg cholesterol.

CHAPTER 5

Be Carb Savvy

These days everyone is talking about "carbs" and whether you should be on a low-carb or high-carb diet. Some carbohydrate intake is important to provide the body and, particularly, the brain with energy, but how much and what kind of carbohydrate is best? To understand this, it is important to know about the various types of carbohydrates.

Simple and Complex Carbohydrates

Carbohydrates are divided into two main types: simple and complex. Simple carbohydrates are sugars, formed by one or two carbohydrate molecules joined together. Simple carbohydrates found in food include fructose (fruit sugar), sucrose (table sugar), and lactose (milk sugar). Complex carbohydrates consist of more than two carbohydrate molecules joined together, and these include starch and fiber.

In the body, most carbohydrates (except fiber) are reduced to a form that the body can use for energy, called glucose, or "blood sugar." Because fiber is not absorbed by the body, it does not contribute to the body's available energy, passing instead through the digestive system to be excreted. Simple carbohydrates are absorbed by the body fairly quickly and so they can elevate the blood-sugar level very rapidly. In fact, simple sugars are the only nutrient that can be absorbed by the tissues inside the mouth because they don't require any digestion. Complex carbohydrates, on the other hand, must be digested in the stomach and pass into the intestines for absorption, allowing the blood sugar to rise more gradually and evenly.

We need to consume both simple and complex carbohydrates, according to our bodies' needs for energy. For example, during exercise, our bodies use energy in the form of glucose at a much faster rate than when we are at rest. Intense exercise is a time that may call for additional consumption of simple carbohydrates. Simple carbohydrates also contribute to the absorption of water in the body and therefore play a vital role in hydration.

CHOOSING CARBOHYDRATES

Most of the time, however, complex carbohydrates are sufficient to meet our bodies' energy needs and tend to be the better choice. Simple carbohydrates are often found in processed foods, snack foods, candy, and sweetened beverages. High consumption of these sugary foods and beverages are known to cause tooth decay and to contribute to the development of unhealthy fats, specifically triglycerides and low-density lipoproteins (LDLs) in the body. Moreover, because sugars are quickly digested and absorbed, they do not contribute significantly to satiety (the sensation of being full and satisfied after a meal), which can lead to overeating.

Most Americans eat too many simple carbohydrates, in the form of sugars, and would benefit from cutting back. The average American consumes more than 267 cups of sugar per year in soft drinks alone! Add this to the amount of desserts, cookies, sugary cereals, candy, and other sugar-laden beverages and snacks, and you can see that as a nation we are consuming too much sugar.

Meanwhile, most people in the United States eat only about two servings a day of fruits or vegetables, which are good sources of complex carbohydrates. Other sources include pasta, rice, bread products, and healthful cereals. When choosing complex carbohydrate products, choose those made with whole grains, such as whole wheat, oats, and rye. Read food labels for carbohydrate content, and choose foods that list lower "Sugars" content as compared with what is listed as "Other Carbohydrate" or starch. Because fiber is not absorbed by the body, it can be subtracted from the "Total Carbohydrate" content when calculating the net carbohydrate provided by the product.

SUGAR SUBSTITUTES

Many people are cutting back on simple carbohydrate intake by using sugar substitutes. There are several good products on the market, which are noncaloric and can even be used in baking. These products include saccharin, aspartame, sucralose, and acesulfame-K. Each of these products has different properties. For example, aspartame breaks down when heated and loses its sweetness, making it unusable for sweetening cooked foods. It is considered safe for all but a very small group of individuals who are unable to properly metabolize

FYI

Vending machines offer chips, candy bars, and regular sodas, which provide lots of calories and very little nutritional value. With a little planning, you can avoid these convenience foods. Buy easy-to-carry healthful foods at the grocery store, and grab what you need in the morning before you start your day.

phenylalanine, one of the two amino acids found in aspartame. Saccharin has been somewhat controversial, with a questionable link to cancer in animals; however, research on this product has not yielded clear results in humans. Sucralose is made from sugar but has been modified so that the body cannot absorb it. It has been used successfully in many products, providing low-sugar alternatives to otherwise sugary foods. Sucralose has been studied extensively over a twenty-year period and been found to be safe for use in foods.

When using alternative sweeteners, it is wise to read up on the cooking and baking recommendations for particular products because they will react differently when heated. The easiest way to do this is to go to a product's website to gather recommendations and even recipes. Once you understand how best to use the products, you can make very tasty low-sugar foods in your own home.

Some sweeteners on the market are not noncaloric. These refer to a type of sugar called sugar alcohols, and they include mannitol, sorbitol, and xylitol. Sugar alcohols are not as sweet as regular sugars and are often used in sugar-free gums and mints. While they are better than regular sugar, they do provide 2 to 4 calories per gram and can cause diarrhea when eaten in large amounts.

FYI

Sucralose is a noncaloric sweetener derived from sugar. It has an excellent safety profile both in the United States and internationally, and it has been cleared for consumption by pregnant and breastfeeding women, as well as children.

REDUCING SUGAR IN OUR DIETS

There are many ways to reduce the amount of sugar in your diet. Switching to diet soft drinks is a great first step, and though it may take some getting used to, your tastes will adjust. Taking time in the grocery store to read labels is another important step. Look for products with low sugar content, and those that use alternative sweeteners to achieve that good taste you are looking for. Try using sugar substitutes for tea, coffee, and when preparing and baking sweet dishes. Once you learn how to use them effectively, you'll hardly notice the difference. You don't have to sacrifice taste to achieve a healthier diet, if you take the time to make the right changes.

Almond Cookies

Almonds are a great way to get antioxidants. They contain polyphenols and vitamin E, as well as fiber. Like most nuts, almonds are high in monounsaturated fats so are best stored in a cool, dry place, or in the refrigerator to prevent the fat from turning rancid.

---

1 cup (225 g) omega-3-rich margarine

1 cup (25 g) sugar substitute

3 egg whites, divided

1 teaspoon almond extract

¼ teaspoon baking soda

2 cups (240 g) all-purpose flour

½ cup (60 g) flaxseed, ground

½ cup (60 g) almonds, halved

In a medium-size bowl, cream margarine and sugar substitute with a mixer until fluffy. Add 2 of the egg whites and the almond extract while beating with the mixer. In a separate bowl, mix together the baking soda, flour, and flaxseed. Gradually blend in with the margarine mixture. Cover and chill in the refrigerator for 2 hours.

Preheat oven to 300°F (150°C, or gas mark 2). Remove dough from refrigerator. Roll into walnut-size balls with your hands. Press the balls flat onto a cookie sheet lined with parchment paper. Press an almond into the center of each cookie. In a small bowl, beat remaining egg white with a fork. Brush the tops of the cookies with beaten egg white.

Bake 15 to 18 minutes. Increase heat to 350°F (180°C, or gas mark 4), and continue baking until golden brown, about 10 minutes.

Yield: About 2 dozen cookies

FYI

Aspartame is an artificial sweetener made from amino acids, making it undesirable for use in baked or cooked products because the amino acids break down with heat and it loses its sweetening power.

Nutritional Analysis: Each cookie provides 138 calories; 10 g fat; 3 g protein; 9 g net carbohydrate; 1 g dietary fiber; and 0 mg cholesterol.

Almond Biscotti

This is a favorite recipe of my Aunt Betty, which I've adapted to increase the omega-3 content. When I first tried it, I was amazed at how easy it is to make biscotti—and how delicious these Italian cookies are!

1½ cups (180 g) all-purpose flour

¼ cup (30 g) ground flaxseed

¼ cup (50 g) sugar

½ cup (12 g) sugar substitute

2 teaspoons baking powder

½ teaspoon cinnamon

¼ teaspoon (72 g) salt

1½ cups (88 g) almonds, roughly chopped

3 egg whites

2 tablespoons (28 ml) plus 1 teaspoon (5 ml) nonfat milk

2 tablespoons (28 ml) canola oil

2 teaspoons (10 ml) vanilla

Four to five 1-ounce (28 g) squares bittersweet chocolate, optional

Preheat oven to 350°F (180°C, or gas mark 4). Line a baking sheet with parchment paper.

Mix flour, flaxseed, sugar, sugar substitute, baking powder, cinnamon, and salt in a large mixing bowl. Mix in the almonds. In a separate bowl, whisk the egg whites, nonfat milk, canola oil, and vanilla. Add to the flour mixture. Knead lightly in the bowl, and transfer to a floured surface. Knead until the dough is smooth.

Divide the dough in half to make two 12-inch (30-cm) long logs. Place the logs on the parchment paper and press down until they are 2-inches (5-cm) wide and 1-inch (2.5-cm) high. Bake 30 minutes. Slide the rolls and the paper onto a cooling rack, and let cool for 30 minutes.

Reheat the oven to 350°F (180°C, or gas mark 4), and line 2 baking sheets with parchment paper. Using a serrated knife, cut the biscotti logs diagonally into ½-inch (1-cm)-wide slices. Place the slices cut-side down on the parchment paper and bake another 10 minutes. (The second baking gives the biscotti its distinctive crunch.) Remove from the oven and cool on the pans.

For a special treat, coat one end of each biscotti with chocolate: Break chocolate into small squares and melt in a double boiler, stirring often. Quickly dip cooled biscotti ends in chocolate and place on parchment paper until chocolate is hardened.

Yield: About 48 pieces

Nutritional Analysis: Each biscotti provides 58 calories; 3 g fat; 2 g protein; 5 g net carbohydrate; 1 g dietary fiber; and 0 mg cholesterol.

All-American Applesauce Cake

This is an old-fashioned recipe that has been modified to make it healthier.
Serve it with a dollop of nonfat whipped topping for dessert,
or by itself as a coffee cake. Leave the skin on the apples because it
contains quercetin, an antioxidant associated with protection against cancer.

½ cup (112 g) omega-3-rich margarine

1 cup (25 g) sugar substitute

1½ cups (450 g) unsweetened applesauce

2 teaspoons baking soda

1 teaspoon ground cinnamon

1 teaspoon ground cloves

1½ cups (180 g) all-purpose flour

½ cup (60 g) whole wheat flour

½ cup (80 g) golden raisins

2 apples, cored and finely diced

1 cup (125 g) walnuts, finely chopped

Canola oil spray

1 tablespoon (6 g) confectioners' sugar, optional

Preheat oven to 350°F (180°C, or gas mark 4).

Melt the margarine and mix with sugar substitute in a large mixing bowl. In a separate bowl, mix together the applesauce and baking soda. Add to margarine mixture, and blend well. Combine cinnamon, cloves, and flours in a small bowl, and add to the margarine mixture. Mix in raisins, apples, and walnuts.

Lightly spray a 9-inch (22.5-cm) square pan with canola oil. Dust lightly with flour. Bake for 40 minutes, until a toothpick inserted in the center comes out clean. Dust lightly with confectioners' sugar, if desired.

Yield: 12 to 14 servings

Nutritional Analysis: *Each serving provides 240 calories; 13 g fat; 5 g protein; 24 g net carbohydrate; 3 g dietary fiber; and 0 mg cholesterol.*

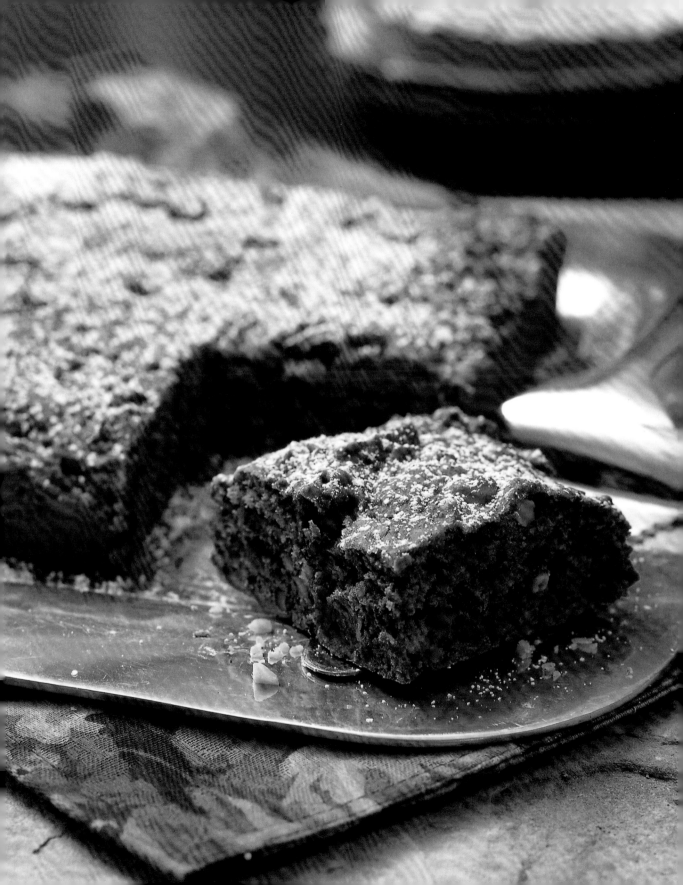

Cherry Walnut Balls

Adding dried cherries to this traditional European treat adds not only a tart-sweet flavor, but also valuable antioxidants, including vitamin A, anthocyanins, and melatonin. Cherries are similar in antioxidant capacity to blueberries and blackberries.

---

1 cup (224 g) omega-3-rich margarine

¼ cup (6 g) sugar substitute

½ teaspoon vanilla extract

2¼ cups (270 g) all-purpose flour

¼ teaspoon salt

1½ cups (88 g) walnuts, finely chopped

½ cup (60 g) dried cherries,
    finely chopped

½ cup (50 g) confectioners' sugar

Preheat oven to 350ºF (180°C, or gas mark 4). In a large bowl, beat together the margarine, sugar substitute, and vanilla until creamy. Slowly stir in the flour and salt until well blended. Stir in walnuts and dried cherries.

Shape into 1-inch (2.5-cm) balls and place on a cookie sheet lined with parchment paper. Bake 13 to 15 minutes, until cookies are lightly browned on the bottom. Remove from oven and set aside for 2 to 3 minutes, until cool enough to handle. Place the confectioners' sugar in a shallow dish. Roll the cookies in the confectioners' sugar while still warm, then set aside to cool.

Yield: About 30 cookies

Nutritional Analysis: Each cookie provides 140 calories; 10 g fat; 3 g protein; 11 g net carbohydrate; 1 g dietary fiber; and 0 mg cholesterol.

FYI
Nearly 60 percent of the average person's sugar intake comes from corn sweeteners, used in high amounts to sweeten sodas and other foods.

Apple Cherry Walnut Pie

My mother used to put red cinnamon candies in her apple pies to add color and flavor. You can use them as substitutes for the ground cinnamon and cloves in this recipe, sprinkling them all around the pie just before adding the topping.

For the crust:

½ cup (60 g) all-purpose flour

½ cup (60 g) whole-wheat flour

¼ cup (30 g) flaxseed, ground

¼ teaspoon salt

½ cup (112 g) omega-3-rich margarine

6 tablespoons (84 ml) cold water

Canola oil spray

For the filling:

5 apples, cored and chopped

1 cup (125 g) dried cherries, chopped

½ cup (12 g) sugar substitute

For the topping:

⅔ cup (80 g) whole-wheat flour

¼ cup (6 g) sugar substitute

¼ cup (55 g) brown sugar

½ cup (60 g) walnuts, chopped

1 teaspoon ground cinnamon

¼ teaspoon ground cloves

6 tablespoons (80 g) omega-3-rich margarine

To make the crust: In a large bowl, mix together the flours, flaxseed, and salt. Mix in the margarine, using a fork to blend, until the mixture resembles coarse crumbs. Sprinkle a little water at a time on the dough, until it is moist enough to form into a ball. Flatten the dough ball on a lightly floured surface, and roll out to about 12 inches (30 cm) in diameter.

Preheat oven to 375°F (190°C, or gas mark 5). Lightly spray a 9-inch (22.5-cm) deep-dish pie pan with canola oil, and sprinkle with flour. Lay the dough into the pie pan.

To make the filling: In a large bowl, stir together the apples, dried cherries, and sugar substitute. Spoon into the pie pan. Mix together the topping ingredients, and pour over the apple mixture.

Bake 50 to 55 minutes, until the top is golden brown.

Yield: 10 to 12 servings

Nutritional Analysis: Each serving provides 330 calories; 20 g fat; 5 g protein; 31 g net carbohydrate; 6 g dietary fiber; and 0 mg cholesterol.

Cherry Blueberry Flambé

Pitting cherries is easy using a cherry pitter, or cherries can be pitted just as easily with a small, curved paring knife. Make a cut around the cherry, and twist the two halves in opposite directions to break apart and expose the pit. With the tip of the knife, carefully thrust out the pit from one half.

½ cup (12 g) sugar substitute

2 tablespoons (16 g) cornstarch

¼ cup (60 ml) cold water

¼ cup (60 ml) orange juice

½ teaspoon orange zest

1 pound (455 g) dark, sweet cherries, pitted

1 pint (300 g) blueberries

1 teaspoon vanilla extract

⅓ cup (80 ml) brandy or kirsch

3 cups (450 g) low-fat frozen yogurt

⅓ cup (50 g) whole almonds, toasted

Mix sugar substitute with cornstarch in a medium-size saucepan. Add cold water and mix until dry ingredients are completely dissolved. Blend in orange juice and orange zest. Bring mixture to a boil over medium-high heat, whisking constantly until it is thickened. Stir in the cherries, blueberries, and vanilla, reduce heat, and simmer 5 to 8 minutes, stirring gently.

Warm brandy in a separate saucepan. When ready to serve, transfer the cherry-blueberry sauce into a decorative casserole dish. Pour the warm brandy or kirsch over the top and ignite. When blue flame goes out, spoon over frozen yogurt in dessert dishes. Decorate with whole almonds, and serve.

Yield: 6 to 8 servings

Nutritional Analysis: Each serving provides 320 calories; 8 g fat; 10 g protein; 44 g net carbohydrate; 3 g dietary fiber; and 55 mg cholesterol.

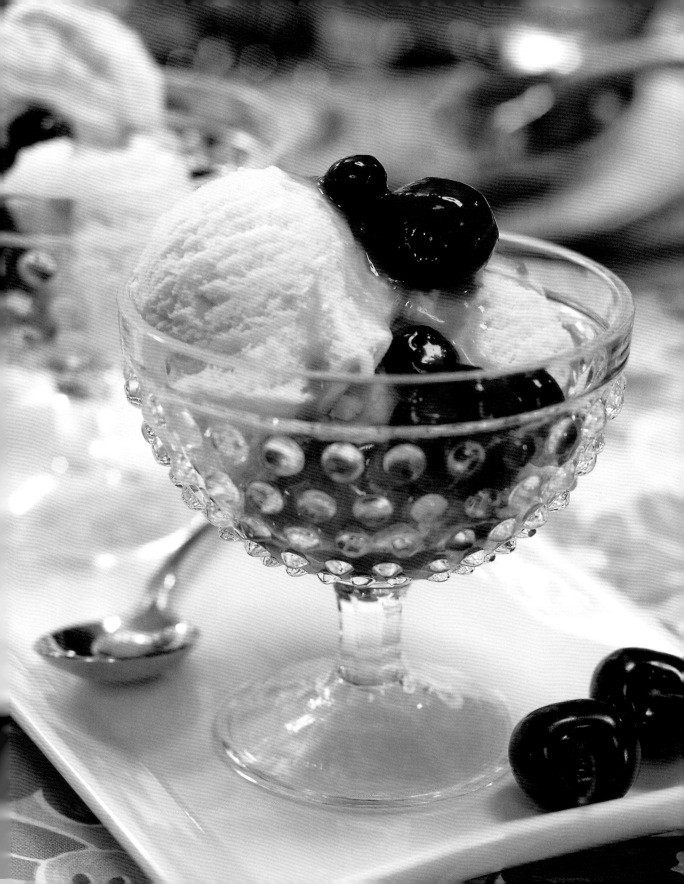

Chocolate Tofu Pudding

Tofu is a high-protein, low-fat food made from soybeans, which contain all of the amino acids essential to human nutrition. Regular consumption of soy protein has been shown to lower the risk of heart disease, so this dish is a much healthier alternative to traditional pudding!

---

6 ounces (170 g) bittersweet chocolate, chopped
¼ cup (30 g) unsweetened cocoa powder
½ cup (120 ml) water

One 16-ounce (455 g) package firm tofu
¼ cup (60 ml) soy milk
1 tablespoon (14 ml) vanilla extract
8 ounces (225 g) fresh strawberries
1 banana

Melt the chocolate, cocoa powder, and water over a double boiler. Set aside to cool.

In a blender or food processor, combine tofu, melted chocolate, soy milk, and vanilla extract. Process until the mixture is smooth and creamy.

Pour into individual pudding dishes, and place in the refrigerator to chill for 1½ to 2 hours.

Slice and quarter strawberries and banana. Serve over pudding.

Yield: 6 to 8 servings

Nutritional Analysis: Each serving provides 210 calories; 9 g fat; 7 g protein; 25 g net carbohydrate; 5 g dietary fiber; and 0 mg cholesterol.

FYI
Cacao beans, used to make chocolate, are one of the richest sources of flavonoids, which help lower blood pressure and maintain a healthy heart. Dairy products, however, interfere with the absorption of the antioxidants in chocolate, so milk chocolate, and dark chocolate consumed along with milk, do not have the protective effects of dark chocolate alone.

Dark Chocolate Strawberry Shortcake

Strawberries contain anthocyanins, which give them their bright red color. Anthocyanins are powerful antioxidants that have been shown to protect cells from oxidative damage. The phenols in strawberries have anti-inflammatory properties. Strawberries are also a great source of vitamin C: One cup provides more than 100 percent of the average adult recommended daily value.

---

2 cups (240 g) all-purpose flour

½ cup (125 g) unsweetened baking cocoa powder, divided

1 cup (25 g) sugar substitute, divided

2 teaspoons baking powder

½ teaspoon baking soda

¼ teaspoon salt

¼ cup (55 g) omega-3-rich margarine

⅓ cup (60 g) miniature chocolate chips

½ cup (120 ml) fat-free half-and-half

¼ cup (60 g) plain nonfat yogurt

4 pints (1.4 kg) strawberries, stemmed and sliced, divided

Nonfat whipped topping

Preheat oven to 400°F (200°C, or gas mark 6).

In a large bowl, mix together the flour, cocoa powder, ½ cup (12 g) sugar substitute, baking powder, soda, and salt. Add the margarine and mash with a fork, until the mixture forms coarse crumbs. Add the chocolate chips, half-and-half, and yogurt. Mix until the dough forms a ball. Place the dough on a lightly floured surface, and knead until smooth. Roll out to about 1-inch (2.5-cm) thick. Using a 2-inch (5-cm) round cookie cutter, cut out 12 to 15 shortcakes.

Line a cookie sheet with parchment paper. Place the shortcakes on the parchment paper and bake for 15 minutes. Remove from oven and set aside to cool.

Place 2 cups (220 g) of the strawberries and remaining sugar substitute in a blender or food processor. Process until smooth. Mix with the remaining strawberries in a medium-size bowl.

Cut the shortcakes in half, place a spoonful of nonfat whipped topping between the 2 halves, and serve topped with the strawberry topping.

Yield: 12 to 15 servings

Nutritional Analysis: Each serving provides 165 calories; 6 g fat; 4 g protein; 23 g net carbohydrate; 4 g dietary fiber; and 1 mg cholesterol.

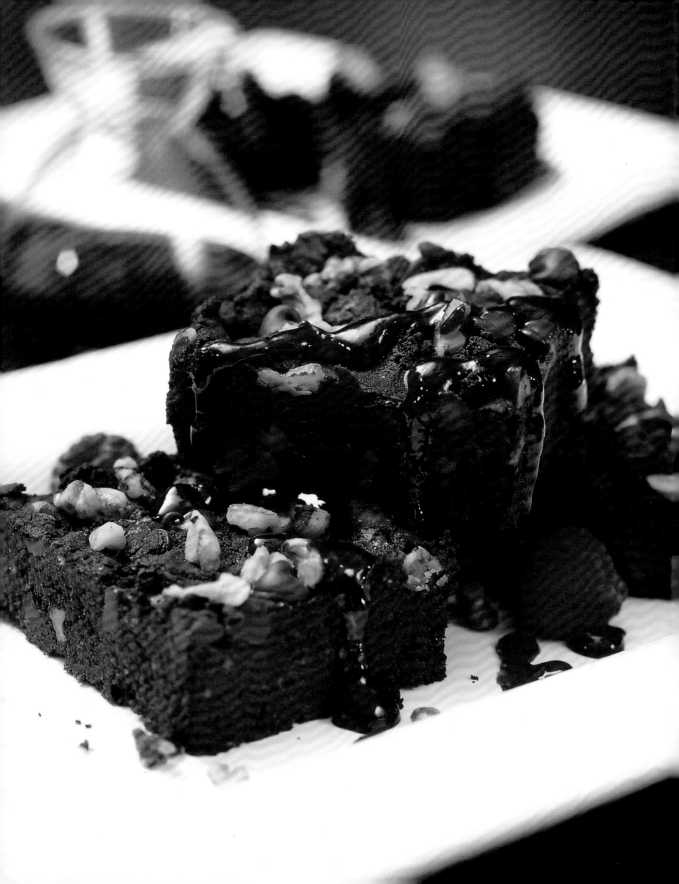

Chocolate Walnut Brownie Indulgence

A clever way to reduce calories in any chocolate recipe is to replace the oil with puréed prunes. The prunes have a chocolaty flavor and are easily found in the baby food aisle of the grocery store.

For the brownies:

Canola oil spray

4 squares (1 ounce [28 g] each) unsweetened chocolate

½ cup (100 g) puréed prunes

3 egg whites

2 tablespoons (28 ml) plus 1 teaspoon (5 ml) nonfat milk

2 tablespoons (28 ml) canola oil

1 teaspoon vanilla extract

¼ teaspoon salt

1½ cups (37 g) sugar substitute

¾ cup (90 g) all-purpose flour, sifted

½ cup (60 g) walnuts, chopped

½ cup (88 g) chocolate chips

For the sauce:

6 ounces (170 g) fresh or frozen raspberries, thawed

⅛ cup (3 g) sugar substitute

1 tablespoon (14 ml) lemon juice

1 tablespoon (14 ml) water

1 tablespoon (14 ml) raspberry-flavored liqueur

For the topping:

1 cup (200 g) nonfat whipped topping, optional

To make the brownies: Preheat oven to 350°F (180°C, or gas mark 4). Spray the bottom of a 9 × 13-inch (22.5 × 32.5-cm) pan with canola oil. Melt the chocolate and puréed prunes in a double boiler, stirring occasionally. Whisk together the egg whites, nonfat milk, and canola oil in a medium-size mixing bowl. Add vanilla and salt. Stir in the sugar substitute and flour, and blend with the chocolate mixture. Add the walnuts and chocolate chips. Spread evenly into baking pan. Bake for 30 minutes. Allow brownies to cool before cutting into squares.

To make the sauce: While brownies are cooking, prepare the sauce by combining all of the ingredients in a food processor or blender. Process until smooth. Drizzle sauce over brownies and top with a dollop of nonfat whipped topping, if desired.

Yield: 16 servings

Nutritional Analysis: Each serving provides 160 calories; 10 g fat; 4 g protein; 12 g net carbohydrate; 3 g dietary fiber; and 0 mg cholesterol.

Fruity Peppernuts

Peppernuts are a traditional European Christmas cookie. In Scandinavia, the cookies are tossed into a roomful of expectant children, who scramble to gather them up. My grandmother kept peppernuts in her candy dish at Christmastime, and I always made sure to get a handful. This recipe is a more healthful version, with added omega-3s and fiber, and is good all year round!

1 cup (225 g) brown sugar

1 cup (25 g) sugar substitute

¼ cup (55 g) omega-3-rich margarine

4 egg whites

1 cup (245 g) yogurt

¼ cup (75 g) unsweetened applesauce

1 teaspoon vanilla

½ pound (225 g) pitted dates, finely chopped

1 cup (125 g) walnuts, finely chopped

1 teaspoon baking powder

1 teaspoon baking soda

2 teaspoons cinnamon

1 teaspoon nutmeg

1 teaspoon allspice

3 cups (360 g) whole-wheat flour

½ cup (60 g) flaxseed, ground

Canola oil spray

Cream together brown sugar, sugar substitute, and margarine. Add egg whites and beat well. Blend in yogurt, applesauce, and vanilla. Stir in dates and walnuts until well mixed. In a separate bowl, mix together remaining dry ingredients. Using a spoon, add small amounts of the dry mixture to the batter, mixing well until a soft dough is formed. Chill overnight in the refrigerator.

Preheat oven to 350°F (180°C, or gas mark 4). Divide dough into 3-inch (7.5-cm) balls. Roll each ball into a rope on a smooth, floured surface. Using a dull knife, cut the rope into ½-inch (1-cm) pieces, about the size of a small nut. Place on a baking sheet sprayed with canola oil and bake 10 to 12 minutes, or until golden brown.

Yield: About 3 cups of mini-cookies

Nutritional Analysis: Each ¼ cup of peppernuts provides 178 calories; 6 g fat; 5 g protein; 25 g net carbohydrate; 3 g dietary fiber; and 0 mg cholesterol.

Dark Chocolate Almond Mousse

My daughter, Bria, loves dark chocolate, so it's not surprising that she came up with this recipe idea. Dark chocolate is thought to contribute to lower blood pressure, and contains flavonoids similar to those found in green tea. For variety, add a thin layer of sweetened coconut on top of the mousse in each cup.

---

6 ounces (170 g) 60-percent cacao
    bittersweet chocolate

Pinch of salt

3 tablespoons (45 ml) hot water

1 tablespoon (15 ml) canola oil

1 tablespoon (15 ml) almond extract

¼ cup (30 g) unsweetened cocoa powder

¼ cup (6 g) sugar substitute

¼ cup (60 ml) nonfat milk

1 teaspoon unflavored gelatin

2 egg whites

1 cup (200 g) nonfat whipped topping

¼ cup (35 g) whole almonds, lightly
    toasted

Melt the chocolate and salt in a double boiler, stirring often. Remove from heat. Add in hot water, canola oil, and almond extract, and blend well. Blend in cocoa powder and sugar substitute. Pour milk into a separate small bowl and sprinkle gelatin over until it absorbs the liquid. Stir milk and gelatin until well blended, and add to the chocolate mixture.

Reheat the chocolate mixture over the double boiler, stirring constantly, until it is completely smooth. Remove from heat and allow to cool to room temperature.

In a small bowl, beat the egg whites until stiff peaks form. With a spatula, carefully fold in the egg whites into the cooled chocolate mixture, combining just until well blended. Do not overmix. Pour the mousse mixture into individual dessert dishes or ramekins, and refrigerate 1 to 2 hours until the mousse is set.

Decorate each serving with nonfat whipped topping and a few toasted almonds.

Yield: 6 servings

Nutritional Analysis: Each serving provides 250 calories; 20 g fat; 6 g protein; 17 g net carbohydrate; 4 g dietary fiber; and 0 mg cholesterol.

FYI
Stevia is a sweetener that has not been approved as a food additive by the Food and Drug Administration, although it may be sold as a "dietary supplement." It is derived from a South American bush.

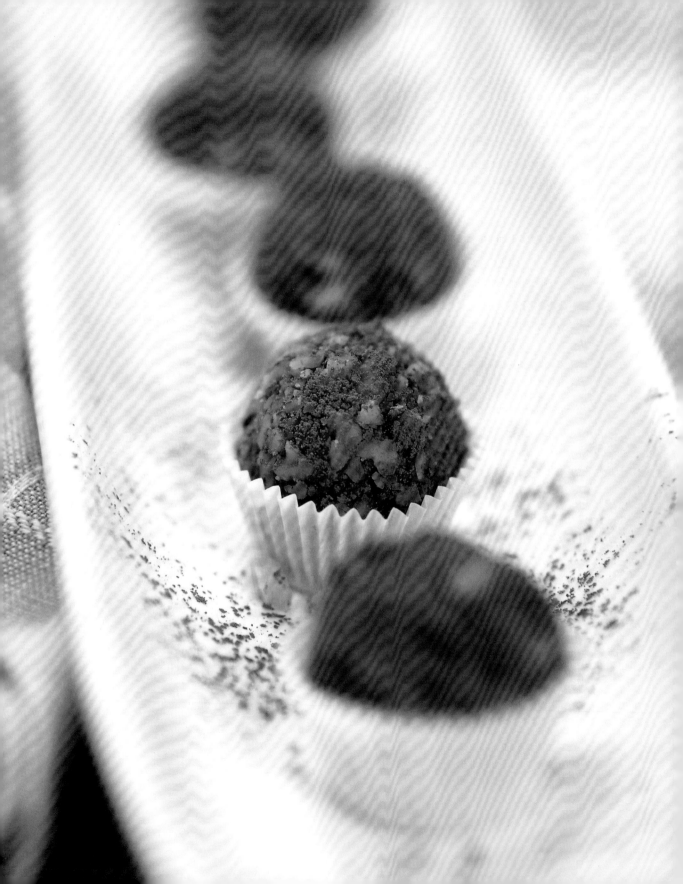

Cranberry-Nut Truffles

Truffles are fun to make and a delightful addition to dinners and parties. For a variation, add a tablespoon (14 ml) of orange liqueur or a teaspoon of cinnamon to the chocolate mixture. Minced candied fruit may be used instead of the dried cranberries. Feel free to experiment!

---

2 cups (350 g) bittersweet chocolate, finely chopped

One 8-ounce (225 g) package fat-free cream cheese

2½ cups (62 g) sugar substitute

1 cup (150 g) orange-flavored, sweetened dried cranberries, finely chopped

2 cups (250 g) walnuts, finely chopped

¼ cup (30 g) unsweetened cocoa powder

Melt chocolate in a double boiler, and set aside to cool. In a large bowl, beat cream cheese until smooth. Gradually beat in sugar substitute. Stir in melted chocolate and dried cranberries, and blend well. Refrigerate 1 to 1½ hours. Place chopped walnuts in a pie pan or shallow dish, and cocoa powder in a second dish. Remove chocolate mixture from refrigerator and shape into 1-inch (2.5-cm) balls, rolling each one in the chopped walnuts first, and then the cocoa powder, until evenly coated.

Store between layers of waxed paper in an airtight container in the refrigerator until ready to serve.

Yield: 36 to 40 truffles

Nutritional Analysis: Each truffle provides 100 calories; 6 g fat; 3 g protein; 9 g net carbohydrate; 1 g dietary fiber; and 0 mg cholesterol.

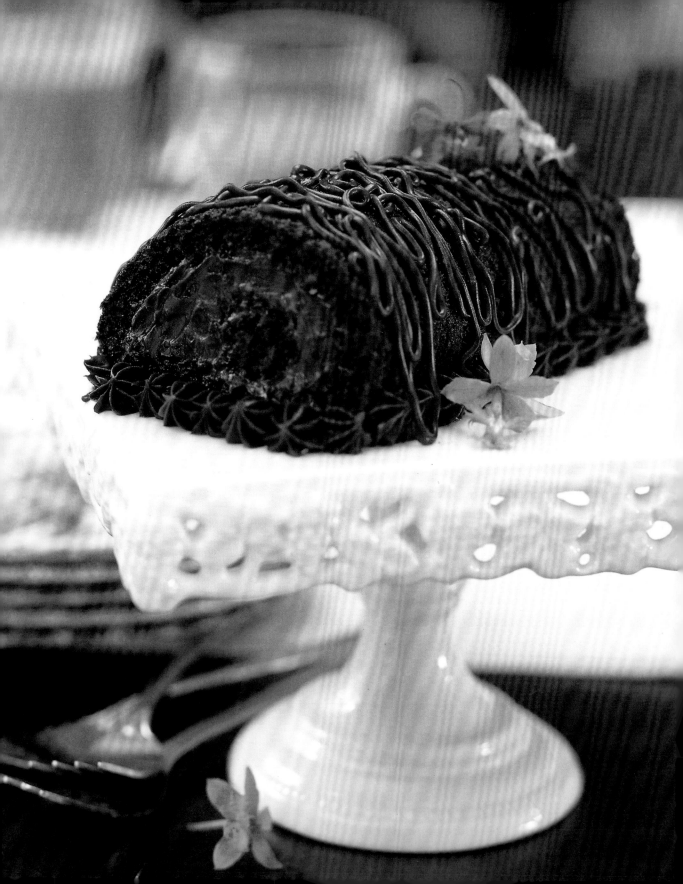

Chocolate Cream Roll

Components of dark chocolate have been associated with lowering blood pressure. In this recipe, nonfat whipped topping can be substituted for the filling. Blend it with the melted dark chocolate and dark chocolate chips.

For the filling:

1 egg white

1 cup (25 g) sugar substitute

3 tablespoons (40 ml) cold water

1 teaspoon cream of tartar

1 tablespoon (15 ml) melted dark chocolate

¼ cup (45 g) dark chocolate, finely chopped, optional

For the roll:

6 tablespoons (45 g) all-purpose flour

6 tablespoons (45 g) cocoa powder

½ teaspoon baking powder

¼ teaspoon salt

4 egg whites

¾ cup (18 g) plus 1 tablespoon (1.5 g) sugar substitute, divided

1 teaspoon vanilla extract

2½ tablespoons (35 ml) canola oil

3 tablespoons (40 ml) soy milk

To make the filling: In a heat-resistant bowl, mix egg white, sugar substitute, cold water, and cream of tartar. Place bowl over a pan of boiling water, and beat with a rotary beater until it stands in peaks. Remove from heat and mix in melted dark chocolate and dark chocolate pieces. Set aside.

To make the roll: Preheat oven to 400°F (200°C, or gas mark 6).

Sift together flour, cocoa powder, baking powder, and salt in a large mixing bowl. In a separate bowl, beat egg whites until stiff. Blend in ¾ cup (18 g) sugar substitute, vanilla, canola oil, and soy milk to egg whites. Stir into flour mixture. Blend well.

Line a shallow 9 × 13-inch (22.5 × 32.5-cm) pan with parchment paper. Pour batter into pan. Bake for 15 minutes. Remove from oven and carefully lift the parchment paper out of the pan. Sprinkle lightly with 1 tablespoon (1.5 g) sugar substitute. Cut off hard crusts. Spread filling evenly over chocolate roll, and roll up. Place on a serving dish, seam side down. Serve sliced.

Yield: 8 servings

Nutritional Analysis: Each serving provides 120 calories; 7 g fat; 4 g protein; 9 g net carbohydrate; 2 g dietary fiber; and 1 mg cholesterol.

Kiwi Pecan Pear Crisp

Kiwifruit are packed with vitamin C and add a tart flavor
to this dish, along with an exotic and colorful flair. In addition,
kiwifruit contain a variety of antioxidants in the form of flavonoids and
carotenoids, and are thought to protect human DNA from oxidative
damage—all compelling reasons to include more of it in our diets!

For the crisp:

8 pears, cored and thinly sliced

¼ cup (40 g) raisins

2 kiwifruit, peeled and quartered

1 tablespoon (14 ml) lemon juice

½ teaspoon lemon zest

¼ cup (30 g) all-purpose flour

¼ cup (30 g) pecans, chopped

½ cup (12 g) sugar substitute

For the topping:

⅓ cup (75 g) omega-3-rich margarine

¼ cup (85 g) honey

1½ cups (112 g) rolled oats

½ cup (60 g) whole-wheat flour

½ teaspoon salt

½ teaspoon ground cinnamon

¼ teaspoon nutmeg

¼ teaspoon cloves

To make the crisp: Preheat oven to 375°F (190°C, or gas mark 5). In a large mixing bowl, combine the pears, raisins, kiwifruit, lemon juice, and lemon zest. Toss gently, and add the flour. Mix the pecans and sugar substitute in a separate bowl, and carefully combine with the pear mixture. Place in a shallow baking dish.

To make the topping: Melt the margarine and honey together. Combine with the remaining topping ingredients and mix well. Spread the topping evenly over the pear mixture. Place dish on the middle rack in the oven. Bake until top is golden brown, about 45 minutes.

Yield: 10 to 12 servings

Nutritional Analysis: Each serving provides 255 calories; 9 g fat; 4 g protein; 38 g net carbohydrate; 6 g dietary fiber; and 0 mg cholesterol.

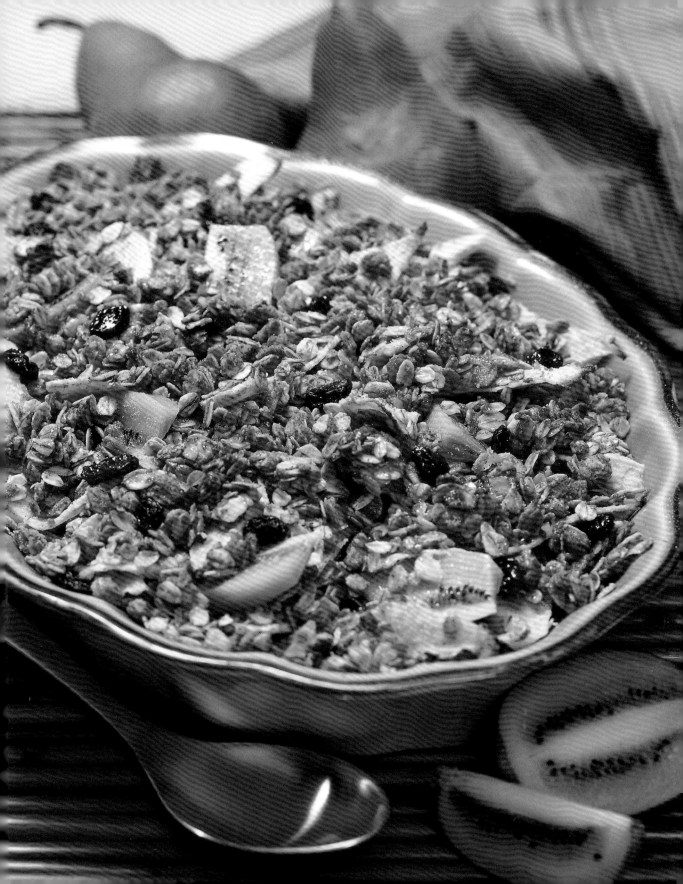

Peach-Berry Port Wine Gelatin

This is a refreshing dish for summer that works with most fruits, so you can substitute your favorites. Avoid using fresh pineapple and papaya because they contain enzymes that will break down the gelatin over time. Use a medium-size to large gelatin mold or individual ramekins for this delicious dessert.

1½ cups (355 ml) pomegranate juice, at room temperature

1 envelope plain gelatin

½ cup (120 ml) water

¾ cup (18 g) sugar substitute

½ cup (120 ml) port wine

1 pint (220 g) fresh raspberries, blackberries, or blueberries

1 cup (110 g) fresh strawberries, sliced

1 to 2 fresh peaches, sliced

Nonfat whipped topping and fresh mint for garnish, optional

Pour pomegranate juice into a small mixing bowl, and sprinkle the gelatin over the top. Do not stir the mixture because this can cause the gelatin to form lumps. Set aside for 5 minutes. Meanwhile, mix together water and sugar substitute.

Set the bowl of gelatin over a pan of simmering water and heat, stirring occasionally, until the gelatin is completely dissolved. Add sugar substitute mixture and port wine. Continue to heat, stirring occasionally, until the liquid clarifies. Pour a thin layer (about ½ inch [1 cm]) of the liquid into a medium-size to large gelatin mold. Chill until set, leaving remaining gelatin at room temperature.

Remove the mold from the refrigerator, and place raspberries and blueberries decoratively on top of the gelatin. Pour enough gelatin over the berries to just cover them. Chill again until set. Remove from the refrigerator and place the peach and strawberry slices alternately on top of the set gelatin. Pour remaining gelatin over the fruit and chill until set.

Remove mold from refrigerator, and place in a container of hot water just below the edge of the mold. Allow mold to sit for 30 seconds before inverting over a serving plate.

Serve as is, or with nonfat whipped topping and mint leaves.

Yield: 8 to10 servings

Nutritional Analysis: Each serving provides 80 calories; 0 g fat; 4 g protein; 12 g net carbohydrate; 2 g dietary fiber; and 0 mg cholesterol.

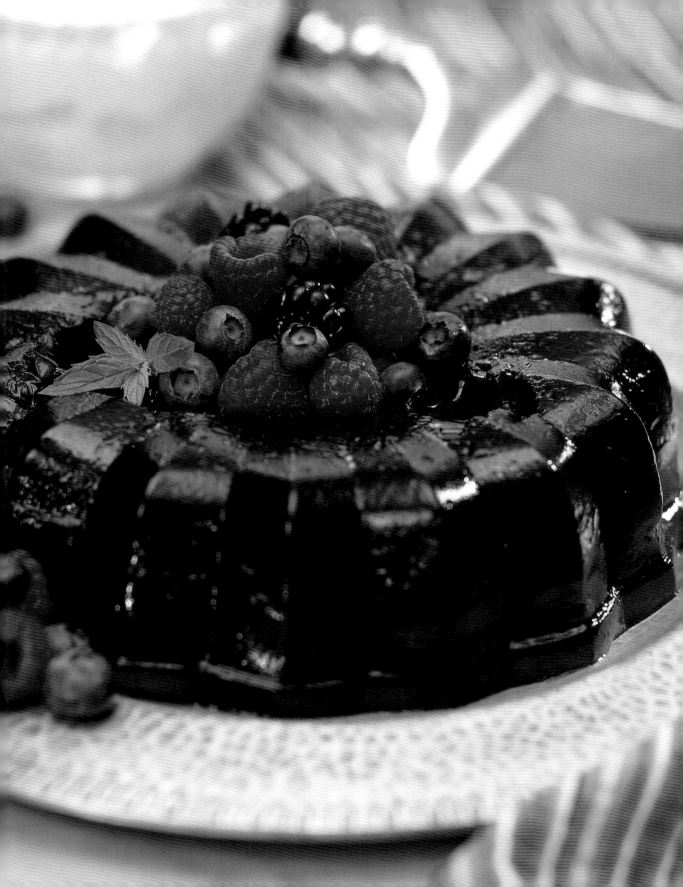

Pecan Cakes with Raspberry Sauce

Walnuts may be used as a substitute
for the pecans as they too are a great source of omega-3s.

For the cakes:

Canola oil cooking spray

¾ cup (75 g) pecans, toasted

½ cup (112 g) omega-3-rich margarine

½ cup (125 g) unsweetened applesauce

1 cup (25 g) sugar substitute

½ cup (100 g) granulated sugar

1 teaspoon vanilla

4 egg whites

2½ teaspoons baking powder

½ teaspoon salt

½ cup (60 g) whole-wheat flour

1½ cups (180 g) all-purpose flour

¼ cup (30 g) ground flaxseed

1¼ cups (295 ml) soy milk

For the sauce:

¼ cup (60 ml) apple juice

1 cup (25 g) sugar substitute

1 tablespoon (8 g) cornstarch

2 cups (220 g) fresh raspberries

1 teaspoon orange zest

Preheat oven to 350°F (180°C, or gas mark 4). Lightly spray and flour 2 muffin or tart pans. Process pecans in a food processor to a medium-fine grind. Set aside.

To make the cakes: In a large mixing bowl, blend margarine, applesauce, sugar substitute, and sugar. Add vanilla and egg whites. In a separate bowl, combine the dry ingredients. Add the pecans and mix well. Add flour mixture and soy milk alternately to the margarine mixture, blending after each addition. Beat the batter on low speed until well blended. Spoon the batter into tart or muffin pans. Bake 15 to 20 minutes, or until a wooden toothpick inserted into the cakes comes out clean. Cool for 5 minutes, and remove from pans.

To make the sauce: Heat the apple juice and sugar substitute in a small saucepan. Once the sauce boils, add the cornstarch, stir well, and turn the heat to low. Simmer 5 to 10 minutes, until the sauce thickens. Remove from heat. Stir in fresh raspberries and orange zest, reserving a few raspberries for the garnish.

Top cakes with raspberry sauce and garnish with fresh raspberries.

Yield: 12 servings

Nutritional Analysis: Each serving provides 280 calories; 15 g fat; 6 g protein; 29 g net carbohydrate; 4 g dietary fiber; and 0 mg cholesterol.

Walnut Bars with Dark Chocolate Drizzle

These great-tasting bars are fun to make on the weekend and can
be stored all week in an airtight container, separated by waxed or parchment
paper. The walnuts, dried cherries, and chocolate are rich in antioxidants,
and using sucralose for the sweetener reduces the calories.

¾ cup (90 g) all-purpose flour

¼ teaspoon salt

1 cup (100 g) walnuts, chopped

1 cup (150 g) dried cherries, chopped

3 egg whites

2 tablespoons (28 ml) plus 1 teaspoon
(5 ml) soy milk

2 tablespoons (28 ml) canola oil

1 cup (25 g) sugar substitute

½ cup (225 g) brown sugar

Canola oil spray

4 to 6 ounces (115 to 170 g)
bittersweet chocolate

Preheat oven to 350°F (180°C, or gas mark 4).

In a medium-size bowl, mix the flour and salt. Add the walnuts and cherries.

In a separate bowl, whisk together the egg whites, soy milk, and canola oil. Add the sugar
substitute and brown sugar, and beat until the mixture is frothy. Fold mixture into flour mixture.

Spray a 9 × 13-inch (22.5 cm × 32.5-cm) baking dish with canola oil spray. Pour in the batter
and place in the oven on the middle rack. Bake until golden brown, about 20 minutes. Remove
and set aside to cool.

Melt the chocolate over a double boiler, stirring constantly, until it is completely smooth.

Cut the bars and place on a sheet of waxed paper. Drizzle each bar with chocolate.

Yield: 12 to 15 bars

*Nutritional Analysis: Each bar provides 190 calories; 9 g fat; 4 g protein; 22 g net carbohydrate;
2 g dietary fiber; and 0 mg cholesterol.*

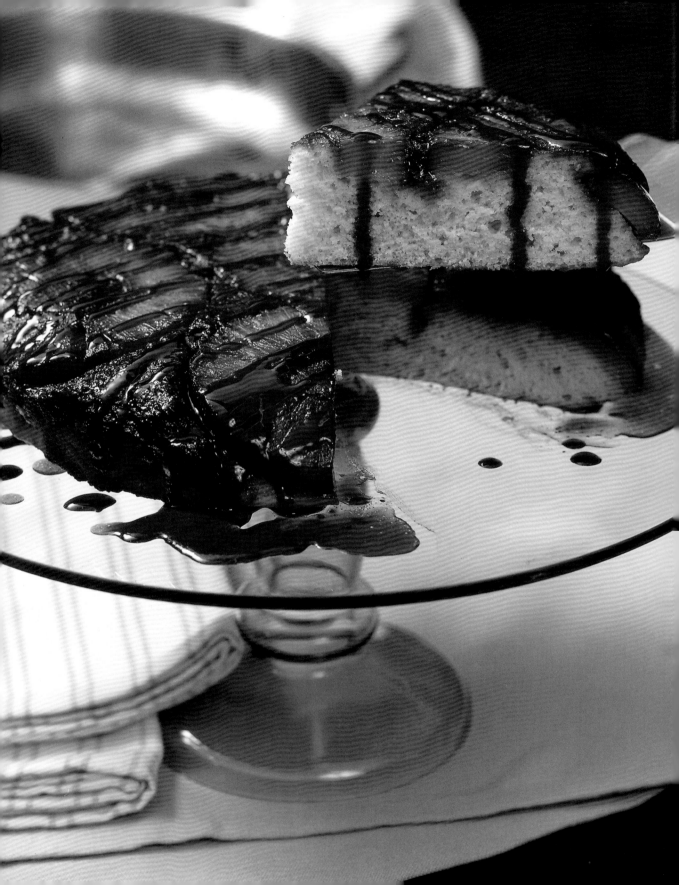

Pineapple Upside-Down Cake

Pomegranate juice, which is used as the sauce for this cake,
has three times the antioxidant power of red wine or green tea.

For the sauce:

One 16-ounce (475 ml) bottle
  pomegranate juice

¼ cup (6 g) sugar substitute

1 tablespoon (8 g) cornstarch

2 tablespoons (28 ml) cold water

For the cake:

3 tablespoons (40 g) omega-3-rich
  margarine

¼ cup (60 ml) molasses

7–8 fresh pineapple slices

3 egg whites

½ cup (120 ml) plus 2 tablespoons (28 ml)
  nonfat milk, divided

3 tablespoons (40 ml) canola oil

1 cup (25 g) sugar substitute

1½ cups (180 g) all-purpose flour

½ teaspoon salt

1½ teaspoons baking powder

Nonfat whipped topping for garnish

To make the sauce: In a saucepan, bring pomegranate juice to a boil. Reduce heat and simmer for about 15 minutes, until the liquid is reduced to 1 cup (235 ml). Stir together the sugar substitute and cornstarch, and make a paste with the cold water. Slowly add the paste to the pomegranate reduction. Cook until sauce is thickened, about 3 minutes, stirring constantly. Set aside.

To make the cake: Preheat oven to 350°F (180°C, or gas mark 4).

Melt margarine and molasses over low heat in a skillet and add pineapple slices. Cook over low heat 3 to 4 minutes.

In a large mixing bowl, whip together egg whites, 2 tablespoons (28 ml) of nonfat milk, and canola oil. Add remaining milk and sugar substitute. Mix well. In a separate bowl, sift together flour, salt, and baking powder. Blend into the egg white mixture, stirring constantly. Pour batter over pineapple slices, place in oven, and bake 45 to 50 minutes.

Remove from oven and invert on a large plate. Serve with pomegranate sauce and nonfat whipped topping.

Yield: 10 servings

Nutritional Analysis: Each serving provides 220 calories; 8 g fat; 4 g protein; 33 g net carbohydrate; 1 g dietary fiber; and 0 mg cholesterol.

Wine-Poached Pears
with Honey-Walnut Sauce

Pears are a good source of vitamin C and copper, which are both important in the antioxidant system. They also contain pectin, a soluble fiber that helps to lower blood cholesterol. Red wine contains a number of antioxidants as well, boosting the benefits of this special dessert.

---

2 cups (470 ml) red wine

2 cups (470 ml) water

1 tablespoon (14 ml) orange juice

1 teaspoon orange zest

1 cup (25 g) sugar substitute

1 cinnamon stick

2 whole cloves

6 firm pears, peeled and halved

Place all ingredients except the pears in a large saucepan. Cook over medium-high heat until the liquid begins to simmer. Reduce heat to low and carefully place the pears in the pan. Simmer for about 10 minutes, turn each half, and simmer another 10 to 12 minutes, until the pears soften.

Gently remove the pears from the pan with a large spoon, and place in a serving dish. Spoon the syrup over the pears. Serve warm or after chilling in the refrigerator.

Yield: 6 servings

Nutritional Analysis: Each serving provides 167 calories; 1 g fat; 1 g protein; 23 g net carbohydrate; 4 g dietary fiber; and 0 mg cholesterol.

FYI
Sugar alcohols are slightly lower in calories than sugar and do not promote tooth decay. These alcohols include sorbitol, xylitol, mannitol, lactitol, and maltitol. They are often used to sweeten sugar-free gum, candies, and cookies, and are considered safe.

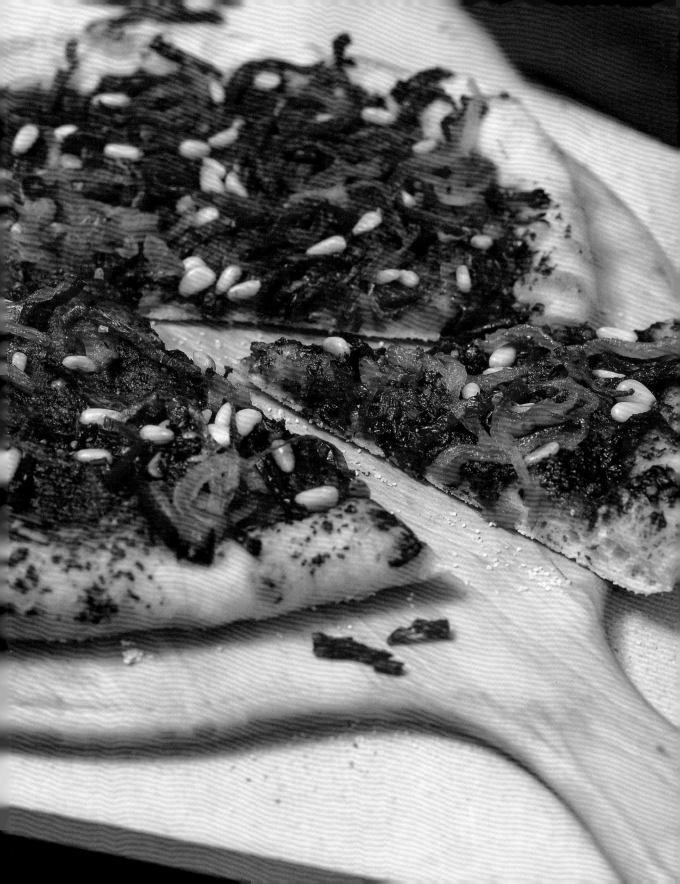

Acknowledgments

I am grateful for my parents, Fran and Paul Hiebert: my mother, an excellent cook, who instilled in me the importance of a well-presented, delicious, and nutritious meal; and my father, himself an accomplished author, who encouraged me to complete this project.

Many heartfelt thanks to my supportive husband, Bryan, and daughter, Bria, who provided ideas and discerning palates for testing many of these recipes. Their love and encouragement, together with my faith, are the primary nutritive elements of my life.

I am also grateful for my nutrition professors at the Loma Linda University School of Public Health, who fueled my passion and gave me the tools I needed to deepen my knowledge of nutrition and food science.

Thanks to all of the Fair Winds Press staff, who assisted me in this project, particularly Amanda Waddell and John Gettings. I am also grateful to Dwayne Ridgaway for his excellent photography and food design.

—Barbara Rowe, M.P.H., R.D., L.D., C.N.S.D.

About the Authors

Barbara Rowe, M.P.H., R.D., L.D., C.N.S.D., has more than seventeen years experience as a dietitian. She has worked individually with countless clients to help them manage their health through diet.

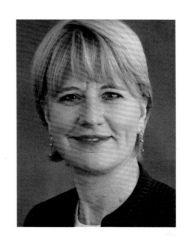

Rowe previously served as program manager for the Johns Hopkins Weight Management Center in Lutherville, Maryland and has authored numerous articles on nutrition. She uses her knowledge of nutrition and her enjoyment of good food to develop great-tasting recipes that promote good health. She lives in Ellicott City, Maryland with her husband, daughter, and three dogs.

Lisa M. Davis, Ph.D., P.A.-C., C.N.S., L.D.N. is a researcher at the Johns Hopkins Bloomberg School of Public Health in Baltimore and Director of Research and Development for Medifast, Inc., a nutritional products company. A former clinician at the Johns Hopkins Weight Management Center, she has been frequently quoted in the popular press, including the *Boston Globe* and *Fitness* magazine, regarding inflammation and diet. Her research includes examining the relationship between brain neurotransmitters and markers of inflammation. She lives in Dayton, Maryland.

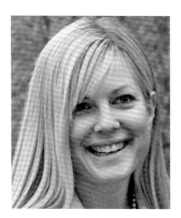

Index